Is Your Cardiologist Killing You?

Sherry A. Rogers, M.D.

Sand Key Company, Inc.
PO Box 19252
Sarasota FL 34276

Is Your Cardiologist Killing You?

Sherry A Rogers, M.D.

Copyright © 2009 by Sand Key Company, Inc.

Sand Key Company, Inc.
PO Box 19252
Sarasota, FL 34276

1-800-846-6687
.prestigepublishing.com

Library of Congress Control Number: 2008910985

ISBN: 978-1-887202-07-7

Printed in the United States of America

Table of contents

Chapter IV
The Mistaken Cases of Heart Failure and Cardiomyopathy

Chapter V
After Your First Heart Attack and/or Stent, You Must
Terminate Progression, Angina, Plaque, and
Coronary Calcifications   **100**

Chapter VI
Solving the Crime   **131**

Books and Services by Sherry A. Rogers, M.D.   **160**

Dedication

God's greatest earthly gift to me, Luscious,
who has continued to grow more luscious over 39 blessed years.
He is infinitely more than the unseen, powerful yet lovingly gentle
"Wind Beneath My Wings".
He is much more than my hero, my idol, my Superman ... my life.

About the Author

Sherry A. Rogers, M.D., board certified by the American Board of Family Practice, is board certified by the American Board of Environmental Medicine, a Fellow of the American College of Allergy, Asthma and Immunology and a Fellow of the American College of Nutrition. She has been in solo private practice in environmental medicine for over 39 years in Syracuse, NY where she sees patients form all over the world. She has lectured at Oxford and in 6 countries where she has taught well over 100 physician courses, has published over fifteen books including the landmark books *Detoxify or Die* and *The Cholesterol Hoax* (www.prestigepublishing.com), over 20 scientific papers, textbook chapters, was environmental medicine editor for *Internal Medicine World Report*, received the American Academy of Environmental Medicine's Dr. Herbert Rinkel Teaching Award for Teaching Excellence, has a referenced monthly newsletter for 20 years, a non–patient consulting service, a lay and professional lecture service, is the guest on over 100 radio shows a year, and more.

Foreword
What Other Doctors Have to Say

After 40 years of brainwashing by the "powers that be", no one was more dedicated to the concept of cholesterol causation of atherosclerosis than was I. I was not only a NASA researcher and an astronaut, but as a medical doctor for 40 years I wrote thousands of prescriptions for whatever cholesterol busters were available. Of course, at that time we had not the slightest awareness of the special needs in our brains for glial cell cholesterol synthesis for memory processing. This knowledge of these specialized brain cells did not surface until much more recently and is now rapidly accumulating. As an example, at the time of this writing well over 1000 reports of transient global amnesia and serious mental disturbance have been reported to Medwatch just from Lipitor alone, since these glial cells are extremely sensitive to statins' touch (http://www.spacedoc.net/662_cases_memory_loss).

Consequently we have one more of many explanations for amnesia, forgetfulness, confusion and disorientation as well as other almost inevitable cognitive side effects that are being overlooked by thousands of physicians. "You're getting older," or, "Perhaps a touch of Alzheimer's?" were the prevailing excuses for this terrible oversight, while the hundreds of cases of the elderly passing on with dementia shortly after statins were started "for their health" is best left buried.

Another of the consequences of the nearly 2 decades of blocking cholesterol synthesis with statin drugs has been the inevitable inhibition of the synthesis of CoQ10, dolichols, selenoprotein, Rho and normal phosphorylation. Unfortunately most doctors have never heard of dolichols, a brain protein closely associated with aggression, hostility, irritability, homicidal ideation, depression, and suicides when they are made deficient by statin drugs. Every thought, every sensation and every emotion you have ever had originates with the synthesis of a specific neuropeptide chain and these are easily damaged by statins by multiple mechanisms. Unfortunately patient claims of bizarre thoughts and actions have been swept under the carpet by many unsuspecting physicians or referred to psychiatry. But the side effects came as no surprise to those of us familiar with the vital role of the mevalonate liver pathway for cholesterol synthesis.

Because the statins also reduce CoQ10 synthesis, which can then lead to far-reaching fatalities, Merck applied for and was granted a patent in May 1990 (US patent office #4,929, 437) for the addition of CoQ10 to their lovastatin (Mevacor). Yet they simply shelved their patent taking no action and somehow completely forgetting to tell the healthcare industry of their special concerns. This oversight has been the direct cause of thousands of other types of statin drug reactions such as peripheral neuropathies, permanent myopathies, chronic disabling neurodegenerative conditions as well as our present concerns about mitochondrial mutations in the very cellular organelles where energy is created.

One dedicated lawyer in this country has filed over 50 Lipitor-associated peripheral neuropathy cases with the courts and he was selecting only the very best from many hundreds of possible cases. My neurologist has decided recently that my statin-associated chronic neuromuscular degenerative process is really primary lateral sclerosis, a close relative of ALS. I have hundreds more ALS-like cases like mine in my repository.

Yet now just recently we have learned that Pfizer is pulling out from statin use right at the end of the over $12 billion profit year with Lipitor. Would any of us as Pfizer executives abandon the most lucrative drug in the history of the world simply because a patent was running out? I wonder exactly what it is. I suspect either the increased cancer incidence of statins (due to their immuno-modulatory effects) or the thousands of cases of nerve and muscle damage now appearing that is associated with statin use. Have they made a decision to back off being associated with statins based on this evidence?

Cholesterol is not public health enemy number one. In fact it is probably our closest biochemical friend. And now, decades after it all began the Enhance and Jupiter/Crestor/CRP studies confirm the complete irrelevance of cholesterol to atherosclerosis: now, how are they going to rationally explain 40 years of the huge cholesterol boo-boo with all the statin damage lawsuits coming down the pike? Jupiter study researchers proved that C-reactive protein (CRP) was one of our best available markers of underlying cardiovascular risk, supporting the earlier Enhance study finding that cholesterol reduction was irrelevant. But because inflammation is a major player in cardiovascular disease and statins are also powerful suppressors of inflammation as well, our priceless mevalonate pathways will continue to be dangerously damaged, ushering new diseases in the unsuspecting patient.

Clearly these statins, as just one example, were "blessed" by the FDA and rushed to market long before their true clinical effects were identified. My head is whirling at the incredible power of our drug companies. Medicine has invented, by recommending drugs to inhibit damaged pathways, a system that bypasses identifying the correctable causes of disease. Meanwhile by turning off cholesterol synthesis, a molecule we cannot live without, we accelerate aging and life-robbing diseases. Dr. Rogers' fine book will help guide you out of this quagmire, into the land where you can find the "cause and cure" of cardiovascular problems.

Duane Graveline, M.D., M PH
Author of *Lipitor, Thief of Memory*, and *Statin Drugs, Side effects, and the Misguided War on Cholesterol*

What you learn is surely a matter of your own life and death. You'll find answers everyone else has missed when you read this book. Dr. Rogers' response to our drug-oriented medical system is to document every provocative statement with uncontroversial and unequivocal proof. Dr. Rogers combines common sense and critical science into a modern medical care package. She is determined to restore health and extend a meaningful lifestyle to as many seriously ill *cardiac cripples* as possible.

Don't be overwhelmed or frightened or discouraged by what you read. Be relieved. Once you see the results no one will be as happy as you and your doctor, because most doctors really do care and want to learn new things that are safe, are evidence-based, and really help. As you will learn, some folks have very simple solutions. Yours could be that simple and you will be on your way to feeling years younger, and able to shed drugs that are destined to create an avalanche of new symptoms. Give your doctor a present of this book and ask if you can work together to correct heart-related nutrient deficiencies and toxicities. Do you have high blood pressure, high cholesterol, cardiac arrhythmias like atrial fibrillation, congestive heart failure or cardiomyopathy or pericarditis? Once you have found the actual underlying causes and cures of your heart disease it no longer matters what your label was.

Doris J. Rapp, M.D.
Author of *Our Toxic World, A Wake Up Call* (www.drrapp.com)
Board Certified in Pediatrics
Board Certified in Allergy
Board Certified Environmental Medicine
Clinical Assistant Prof. (emeritus) of Pediatrics at SUNYAB

Dr. Sherry Rogers is one of the foremost pioneers in the emerging era of environmental medicine. Using her own history of triumphant recovery from prolonged suffering and multiple 'incurable' diseases as well as her meticulous scrutiny of the medical literature, she has relentlessly challenged the existing clinical paradigm of drugs and surgery as the most effective solution to health problems. She has consistently highlighted the need to identify and repair the underlying causes of health afflictions through well-researched strategies and novel interventions in order to heal what is often considered 'the impossible.'

Recognizing that the process of updating the medical model has always been notoriously slow and that countless suffering people do not have time to wait for the lethargic adoption of innovation, Sherry has been candid in her lectures, forthright in publications, and outspoken in media presentations. She has courageously exhorted medical practitioners to collate their medical experience with new and exciting information emerging from scientific research, rather than simply adhering to the status quo.

Her passion and enthusiasm for facilitating the process of advancement and change in the health profession has earned her enormous respect from many colleagues. I encourage health providers and individuals to read Dr. Rogers' recent publications with an open mind and critical thought. Readers will be rewarded with a voluminous amount of invaluable and referenced health information -- -- knowledge that may be life-changing for them and their loved ones.

Stephen J. Genuis, M.D., FRCSC, DABOG, DABEM, FAAEM
Clinical Associate Professor
Faculty of Medicine
University of Alberta

Solving the Crime of Your Stolen Life

Heart disease has become the number one stealth killer in the U.S. But how could this happen with the world's most expensive and high tech medical system? Since victims of heart disease are usually not molecular biochemists, I've created a format here that should make learning easier and a lot more fun. I'll pattern the solution of this mystery after the who-done-it Agatha Christie murder mystery, *Arsenic and Old Lace.*

Here's what you'll learn from cases of hypertension, hypercholesterolemia, arrhythmia, heart failure, cardiomyopathy, angina, coronary artery plaque and other heart maladies:

1. **The mysterious crime** is that folks are needlessly dying from totally curable heart problems. Instead they are being drugged, which leads to further and even more rapidly fatal medical problems, again treated only with drugs.
2. **The clues to curing** versus drugging your symptoms.
3. **The forensic evidence**, and the rest of the evidence from some of the most respected medical authorities and journals.
4. **As well as how to interrogate and cross examine the suspect**, your cardiologist.
5. And I'll show you how to **solve the mysterious crime**. Do you need the help of crime investigators, a PI or police? No. Because the definition of malpractice is merely that you're not doing what the rest of your colleagues are doing. It is not a measure of what is best for the patient, but of conformity.
6. But take heart, for you will end with enough evidence to **make your verdict and decide who is guilty** and who is innocent of one of the best-kept secret crimes of the century.
7. Best of all, you will be protected against further crimes, having been empowered to heal yourself, in spite of the perpetrators.

Introduction

Forty years ago in medical school, I believed cardiologists were the most awesome of doctors. How they could pull so much information out of the squiggles on an EKG, how they skillfully manipulated their pharmacologic knowledge of some of the most potent drugs in the *PDR*, and how they came to the rescue of a patient in the throws of his first heart attack or pulled out all the stops for the aged woman barely able to speak because of heart failure were inspiring.

Then in this era they only got better. They paired up with the cardiovascular surgeons to transplant blood vessels from the legs into hearts. Having a by-pass patient on the heart-lung machine required even more knowledge. Next a quantum leap was made when doctors who basically had elected not to be surgeons were suddenly in the arena at first just doing heart catheterizations, but morphing later into a major "hands-on" specialty of putting in stents. Thus the invasive cardiologist was born and had split off from the non-invasive guy. Meanwhile, billion-dollar a year drugs like Lipitor® and Plavix® gave new meaning to the phrase "blockbuster drug", while stents were inserted at an unprecedented rate. So far, so good. Millions owe their lives to these men and women cardiologists.

But something dangerously bad happened in the process. And millions more lives have been lost and continue to be needlessly lost. So what was so bad? What got lost in the process of this modernization of the field of cardiology? **They forgot to show folks how to heal**. They got so hooked on the glamour of the quick fixes of drugs and surgery that they neglected to show folks that the majority can heal without all this.

In fact they must. For the scariest problem is that for every drug and procedure, there is an unseen but very real downside of not only (1) getting worse more quickly and thereby needing more drugs until drugs no longer work, but also (2) avalanching into an abyss of new and seemingly unrelated, often "incurable", medical problems, including other heart problems, cancer, accelerated ageing and death. **The mystery is how did we allow this to happen**, and who is at fault. More importantly, how are we going to solve this?

Because I don't want one of those premature deaths to be yours, or that of someone dear to you, I have written this book. It is my hope that you will lovingly share it with your cardiologist, for remember, he is pedaling as fast as he can. We have built the medical system for failure, starting with the average 7-minute office visit right on up to an inexperienced insurance clerk determining your medical fate by deciding what you can afford. As *The Wall Street Journal* tells us, the average time a physician spends listening to his patient before he interrupts with a drug treatment is now reported to be 18 seconds. **Every symptom becomes an immediate deficiency of the newest high-priced drug.**

Furthermore, as practicing physicians, we used to go to continuing medical education courses with the sole purpose of learning what was new in medicine. Now many professionals are too busy going to courses to learn how to fill out insurance forms and properly CPT code your procedure so they can get paid. It is this cookie-cutter form of medicine that has taken the joy and purpose out of medicine.

The body's chemistry was miraculously designed to overcome the most devastating atrocities, as I'll show you. **When all that high-tech medicine has to offer has failed, the body has been healed**. But medicine has conveniently jumped right over the education/healing phase in place of office speed and pharmaceutical intervention. My goal here is not to denigrate the cardiologist, but instead allow you to become an important force in bringing him into the real 21st century of molecular cardiology where we physicians teach folks how to heal their bodies. Then when all else fails, cardiologists are there to come to the rescue. Even then, the odds of their heroic rescue being successful are vastly improved because of the efforts you will have learned about here and adjustments you will have made.

So what makes me so smart? I was not at the head of my medical school class. As the oldest of eight in a family where no one had ever graduated from high school, there was no money for college, much less medical school, much less for a female in the sixties. I had to work as well as study. After graduation, I was blessed with over 20 "incurable" maladies. I quickly learned the painful lesson that drugs were not going to cure me, nor were any of my colleagues at the medical school from which I graduated. They were powerless. This forced me to learn what we were not taught in medical school: how to heal the body and not just bludgeon every symptom with a drug, or when that fails, just cut out the part and throw it away.

So if this information is so vital, why doesn't the average cardiologist know and use it? I think you will discover the answers as you read through here. But one clue came right from the famed *New England Journal of Medicine* when they showed that **over 87% of physician "experts" who make the rules or guidelines for medical treatments just happen to benefit financially (in diverse ways, funding research, lectures, being a highly paid consultant, etc.) from the pharmaceutical companies** (Choudhry). Countless other studies show that there is enormous conflict of interest throughout medicine as financial sponsorship of a study has a strong bearing on the positive outcome being in favor of the sponsor (Kjaergard, Als-Nielsen).

And because this information I am about to give those who are totally uneducated in healing the body naturally could be considered controversial, I have documented every statement. That means there is a scientific report from medicine's own medical journals that verifies what I have said. One terrific reason I am able to put this information into such a smaller and handier book is that this book follows my other books, totaling thousands of medical references. Since my goal is now to empower a larger audience, especially folks who never considered themselves as key to healing their own bodies, I have condensed much of the material, relying on the old 80-20 rule: most of the folks or 80% of them will get better with only 20% of what we have to offer.

So for new references or ones I think are particularly important, you will find the author's last name in parentheses. For the backup for all other statements, and for further details on what is here and more protocols for healing that are not in here, including thousands of references that back up all that is said in this book, you may want to start with *Detoxify or Die*, then progress to *The High Blood Pressure Hoax* (even if you do not have high blood pressure since the health of your heart and brain vessels is crucial to the cure and prevention of every disease), then go to *The Cholesterol Hoax*. Again, this is for you even if you do not have high cholesterol, because **cholesterol is a key ingredient in healing the heart, plus the protocols are also the perfect anti-ageing arsenal**. Read these in that order. Our monthly referenced newsletter of 20 years fills in the blanks and keeps you abreast of newer findings. In fact, our readers are continually sending me articles touted as the latest findings in the newspapers and laughingly recalling when they first learned about it 10-15 years earlier in our *Total Wellness* newsletter.

And last, am I just another health-nut out to make a buck? No. I have a completely wonderful life with Luscious and do not rely on these writings. It is a much stronger calling to tear me away from my retirement. At 66 I am completely healthy (having cured over 2 dozen incurable maladies), play two hours of tennis a day and have no symptoms and take no medications. And with all my friends retired, I have enormous enticement to leave all this behind after a successful 39 year career in medicine. Plus I had suffered enough. My severe chemical sensitivity required me to rent oxygen on wheels to deliver lectures, with colitis I filled the toilet bowl with blood 8 times a day between patients, totaled 5 cars due to toxic encephalopathy, and damaged my back 6 times and wore a fiberglass cast so tight that it gave me hemorrhoids, hiatus hernia and varicosities, had amnesia, arthritis, asthma, migraines, eczema, 12 breast fibroadenomas, petit mal seizures, unwarranted depression, MCL knee blow-out, a uterine fibroid, atrial fibrillation and near lethal ventricular tachycardia, a paralyzed leg for 6 weeks, and much more. I thought I had joined the disease-of-the-month club!

Clearly I have an obligation to fulfill. During this chaos, I was steadily forced to learn how to heal, and all without surgery or medications. I suddenly realized that all along it was God's plan. There is no way I should have been a doctor. The odds were against me, as most of the guys in my class came from money, or had dads who were docs, and didn't have to balance their studying with working during med school. No, *I had to be brought to my knees, literally, to the depths of despair in order to learn what I should have been taught in medical school.* And now out of gratitude for having been shown that **God designed the body to heal against all odds**, I need to share this information and teach others how to empower themselves, *even when medicine appears to have given up.*

You will see that if you have been merely managed with drugs, that you are destined to get worse. So where do all these "secret" facts come from? The thing I find the oddest is that **all this information comes from the leading cardiology and other medical and molecular biochemistry journals. It has been right under our noses all along**, sometimes for decades, and continues to emerge. No, I have no anger, especially when I reflect on the thousands of researchers who made all this possible. Each has dedicated his/her life to enlarging our understanding of one more small, but crucial part of the big puzzle we call human health.

Back on the old 80/20 rule, for each cardiac diagnosis that heads a new chapter, I have given just a smattering example of a couple of the top items that have enabled folks to be pleasantly surprised that they could start to reverse their disease, even though they had been to the best of cardiologists. But because the underlying causes and cures of all types of heart disease (and all types of diseases) have so much chemistry in common, let me remind you to keep two things in mind. (1) Read all of this, even if you do not have the diagnosis that heads the chapter, for this entire book is about the health of your heart and its vessels and nerves (and those of every organ of your body). (2) If you do not completely heal yourself, please go to the other books until you do get yourself completely well, vivacious, and off drugs. For that is real health.

I'm not here to put the cardiologists out of business, but to empower you to get the best treatment and find the ultimate cure for your heart symptoms, not just have you fuel the drug industry with an unending avalanche of symptoms that inevitably occurs once you have started on even one drug. **Medicine is stuck in a web that excludes cure for the sake of pharmaceutical profits. And most cardiologists are unknowingly or knowingly entwined in this web. Because many are clueless that there is a world of cure just waiting for them** to take charge, you are given questions you can surreptitiously ask in order to test their knowledge. For you need to clearly know where the guy you have placed in charge of your life stands. I have consulted on and reversed some of the most severe cardiac cases that were resistant to everything modern medicine has to offer. And what blew my mind repeatedly was that it made absolutely no difference if they had been treated by cardiologists in some of the world's most famous clinics and medical centers or by the doc down the street. For we have cloned medical teams to focus on drugs and surgery.

One thing to remember about the pharmaceutical industry is that their mission is to produce drugs. That is what they do. The problem is that suppressing symptoms is not solving medical problems.

But as you will learn, **God has designed the body to heal**. And you will learn how to use natural tools with which to do it. Are you ready to solve a most important mystery of why your chance of dying of heart disease, whether male or female, tops the list? **Are you ready to solve the mystery and prevent yourself from becoming its next victim?** If so, **welcome to the first day of the rest of your life. Let your empowerment begin**.

References:
• Choudhry NK, et al, Relationships between authors of clinical practice guidelines and the pharmaceutical industry, *Journal of the American Medical Association*, 287; 5:612-17, Feb 6, 2002
• Kjaergard LL, et al, Association between competing interests and authors' conclusions: Epidemiological study of randomized clinical trials published in the BMJ, *Brit Med J*, 325-249, 2002
• Als-Nielsen B, et al, Association of funding and conclusions in randomized drug trials, *Journal of the American Medical Association*, 290:921-8, 2003

Chapter I

The Case of High Blood Pressure

The Mystery of the Diuretic Debacle

Now how in the world could your cardiologist be killing you if you merely have high blood pressure? The answer is: Slowly, but very steadily. He probably started you on a diuretic or fluid pill. It is simple plumbing. Lower the pressure in a closed system by letting out some of the fluid and the pressure goes down. It sounds good enough, and the hydrochlorthiazide (HCT) and other diuretics are often cheap. So what could be the problem?

Let's look at the other effects of fluid pills. **Diuretics cause the body to lose the minerals, potassium and magnesium.** When you are low in potassium it leaves you weak, tired and irritable. But **low potassium can also be the very cause of high blood pressure in the first place**. Sometimes something as simple as a diet high in potassium, as in fresh fruits and vegetables can fix that. And carrot juicing a couple of times a day speeds the recovery.

But another major cause of high blood pressure is spasm of the microscopic muscles that surround blood vessels. It is simple. When the muscles that wrap around the blood vessels tighten, the pressure in the "pipes" or blood vessels goes up. **Vessels spasm when they are low in magnesium**. So already you see that the very use of **a diuretic may actually make you get worse**, since it accelerates the loss of minerals whose deficiency may have caused your high blood pressure in the first place. The scientific/medical literature is full of examples of how just giving potassium or magnesium has cured the high blood pressure of many folks. But it gets worse. Let's look more closely at the magnesium clue.

The average diet gives you far less than half of the magnesium that you need in a day, so most folks are low in magnesium to begin

1

with. That is one reason why high blood pressure is so common and *plagues one in four adults*. In fact, a lot of other medical epidemics could be fixed with merely taking magnesium. These include anything with a spasm component, like back muscle spasms mimicking a herniating disc, migraine, spastic colon, asthma, cystitis, depression, angina, and more. Your blood pressure is no exception. And since magnesium also controls the flexibility or fluidity of the cell membrane, its deficiency also contributes to the "leaky" blood vessels and fluid retention in ankles of folks with high blood pressure or heart failure (Rayssiguier). And there are many other nutrients that do this.

In numerous studies well **over half the population is low in magnesium,** and these studies looked at the inferior magnesium, not the one that shows the higher and truer percentage of it. More modern studies show **the American average diet only gives less than one-tenth of the magnesium folks need** (Nielsen). So as you see, **the very drug that is prescribed as first line treatment causes you to lose more magnesium, so your pressure eventually goes higher and requires more drugs**.

Evidence:
- Rayssiguier Y, Magnesium and lipid metabolism. In Sigel H, Sigel A (eds), *Metal Ions in Biological Systems, Vol 26, Compendium on Magnesium and Its Role in Biology, Nutrition and Physiology*, NY: Marcel Dekker, pp341-58, 1990
- Nielsen, see Chapter III

The Clue of the Magnesium Miracle

If your doctor wants, he can measure your magnesium, but don't let him use the wrong test. **Your lab result must say RBC (red blood cell) or erythrocyte magnesium**. If it just says "magnesium", he has ordered the wrong test and it can look "normal " even when you are so low you could have a heart attack in the next minute. For **low magnesium also can cause spasm of the coronary arteries and a heart attack with sudden death**. And you can appreciate that since magnesium deficiency is so common and is a common cause of high blood pressure, that taking a diuretic that makes you lose more magnesium through the urine, sooner or later causes your pressure to go up even higher. You will eventually require another medicine. That is if you don't die of sudden cardiac arrest from low magnesium first!

Sadly this information about magnesium is over a quarter of a century old (Resnick). The mystery is why is it still unknown by the specialists? This poor researcher, Resnick, for example, published a paper on the importance of magnesium in 1984 in a very prestigious journal, and was still doing it in 1997, and now over a decade later cardiologists still do not check magnesium! Go figure.

Start taking one tablespoonful of **Natural Calm** twice a day. If it gives you diarrhea, cut back and fill in with **Chelated Magnesium** up to 3 capsules twice a day, remembering that for many forms the body absorbs only half of the stated amount. Unfortunately all types of magnesium are not equally absorbed. The most potent form requires a prescription, **Magnesium Chloride Solution 200 mg/cc** (windhampharmacy.com). Take ½ teaspoon twice a day (your doctor can learn all about how to write the prescription with the evidence for its necessity in *The High Blood Pressure Hoax*). Whatever combination of magnesium types you choose, get bare minimum 1000 mg a day.

Meanwhile the diuretic raises the blood level of a damaging amino acid, **homocysteine, that is four times more potent a predictor of early heart attacks than a high cholesterol is**. So the guy who prescribes a diuretic without first finding the cause of your high blood pressure and curing it is making sure that *the sick will get sicker, quicker*. At least he should have started with (1) an RBC magnesium, bare minimum. And once he prescribed a diuretic then (2) he should at least have checked your homocysteine level to see if he has put you at even higher risk of an early heart attack. And this is only the beginning. The current standard of care gets far worse.

Evidence:
- Resnick L, et al, Intracellular free magnesium in erythrocytes of essential hypertension: relation to blood pressure and serum divalent cations, *Proc Natl Acad Sci USA,* 81:6511-15, **1984**
- Resnick LM, Magnesium in the pathophysiology and treatment of hypertension and diabetes mellitus: Where are we in **1997**? *Am J Hypertens,* 10:368-70, 1997
- Touyz RM, Role of magnesium in the pathogenesis of hypertension, *Mol Aspects Med,* 24; 1-3:107-36, 2003
- Schimatschek HF, et al, Prevalence of hypomagnesimia in an unselected German population of 16,000 individuals, *Magnes Res,* 14; 4:283-90, 2001 (over 58% were low in magnesium even using the inferior assay)
- Altur BM, et al, Magnesium deficiency in hypertension, *Science,* 223:1315-17, 1984
- Whang R, *J Am Med Assoc,* June 13, 1990 (cited later, over 54% were low in magnesium using an inferior assay)
- Widman L, et al, The dose dependent reduction in blood pressure through administration of magnesium: a double blind placebo controlled cross-over trial, *Am J Hypertension,* 6:41-45, 1993
- Laurant P, et al, Physiological and pathophysiological role of magnesium in the cardiovascular system: implication in hypertension, *J Hypertens,* 18:1177-91, 2000

Never the Suspect,
Always the Hero

To summarize so far, diuretics cause serious wasting of magnesium and potassium. These in turn cause higher blood pressure, arrhythmias, and fatal sudden cardiac arrest. But who suspects the cardiologist? He's the hero who heals your blood pressure. Besides wasting minerals that could have been the cause and cure of your blood pressure, **diuretics** do something worse. They **raise your homocysteine level**. It has been known for decades that when a medicine uses up enough nutrients to raise your homocysteine, it makes you a target for early heart disease. But that is the reason you are treating your blood pressure in the first place --- to prevent heart disease!

The Mystery of Accelerated Aging

If that were not enough, **elevated homocysteine also speeds up getting Alzheimer's, cancer, macular degeneration** (the number one cause of blindness over the age of 50) and other diseases of aging. In fact, you want your homocysteine measured even if you are not on a diuretic, because lots of other things can cause it. Furthermore, **diuretics increase your chances of getting diabetes, losing zinc** (which then promotes a dozen diseases including cancer), and much more.

So far this is not too good, is it? **The number one drug category for treating high blood pressure actually guarantees you will get worse** and not only eventually have higher pressure, but get other medical problems along the way that you might never have blamed on the medication, prescribed by your cardiologist.

Meanwhile, by being on a diuretic that depletes potassium and magnesium, you will eventually need another medication. Sometimes next is often the category of calcium channel blockers, like Norvasc® as one example (see *The High Blood Pressure Hoax* for the other dozens of brand names). In fact before cholesterol-lowering drugs, this was the number one category of heart drugs prescribed by cardiologists.

Calcium channel blockers do just that: block or poison the channels that let calcium into the cell. Again it sounds like a good thing when the medicine stops your high blood pressure. But at what price? Physicians showed that **when a person has been on a calcium channel blocker for just under 5 years, his brain has shrunken away from the skull and his I.Q. drops** considerably (Heckbert). It causes brain rot. He becomes dumber. There is also a higher amount of cancer and heart attacks among folks who take calcium channel blockers, as there should be (Fitzpatrick, Psaty, Bonnet). That's because no one actually fixed the broken calcium channels. **When you don't find and fix what was broken that**

caused high blood pressure, then the damage progresses to create other diseases, including accelerated aging and cancer.

The Clue of the Membrane Oil Change

What damages calcium channels, and what are they anyway? They are pores that permeate the cell envelope or capsule (also called the cell membrane). When cell membranes are finally lacking enough of the crucial nutrients they need, they stop working properly and the calcium pores (channels) leak. Sometimes the repair is incredibly simple. We merely put back the fatty acids that became deficient over the years. Let's look at a common example.

You can often repair the calcium channels with what I call *an oil change*. Start by taking the very **ingredients that repair damaged cell membranes**, which house the broken calcium pores. Putting in new oils (fatty acids) can often fix the chemistry. The most commonly low are EPA and DHA, found in cod liver oil. But in order to repair the membrane, you also need the "innards", made of phosphatidyl choline (Smaby). You can accomplish this sophisticated task quite easily by using a tablespoonful each of **Cod Liver Oil** and **PhosChol** a day for 3-6 months, and then reduce them to 1 teaspoon each. Also important are two **E Gems Elite** twice a day. Don't worry, I'll teach you more about this as we roll along.

However, **it makes no sense to put good oils in the cell membranes to repair the broken calcium channels if you continue to eat the bad oils that caused the damaged calcium channels to begin with**. Trans fatty acids are in most processed foods (even often, as you will learn later, in foods that sport a label on the front of the package saying "*No trans fats*"). So out goes anything with hydrogenated oils. Cook with olive oil or butter, eat no processed foods with hydrogenated or partially hydrogenated (trans fat) oils in them.

Now if you are not concerned enough about your blood pressure to assay and correct your fatty acids, remember that you only have two eyes and preserving your vision depends heavily on the blood vessels in the back of the eye, the retina. Macular degeneration is the leading cause of blindness in folks over 50. Among the many important nutrients to prevent and more importantly reverse it (as many of us have done, even though ophthalmologists ignore it), are the fatty acids (Hodge). And other nutrients you will learn about here to reverse high blood pressure also have a role in preserving the vessels of the eye, like vitamin D (Parekh).

So even if you do not have high blood pressure, you need to know about all this. And not to really overload you with facts, but another reason is that fats like cod liver oil actually "talk" to your genes that regulate every process in your body (Price).

And yes, still take your magnesium, because, guess what? **Magnesium is nature's calcium channel blocker** (Iseri)! So if you've been put on a calcium channel blocker for hypertension or other heart problems such as angina or congestive heart failure without so much as an RBC magnesium and fatty acid assay, that's a serious omission. More on these later.

Evidence:

- Iseri LT, et al, Magnesium: Nature's physiologic calcium blocker, *Am Heart J,* 108; 1:188-192, 1984
- Hodge WG, et al, Evidence for the effect of omega-3 fatty acids on progression of age-related macular degeneration: A systematic review, *Retina,* 27; 2:216-21, 2007
- Parekh N, et al, Association between vitamin D and age-related macular degeneration in the Third National Health and Nutrition Examination Survey, 1988 through 1994, *Arch Ophthalmol,* 125; 5:661-69, 2007
- Smaby JM, et al, Phosphatidylcholine acyl unsaturation modulates the decrease in interfacial elasticity induced by cholesterol, *Biophys, J* 73:1492-1505
- Price T, et al, Omega-3 polyunsaturated fatty acid regulation of gene expression, *Curr Opin Lipidol,* 11:3-7, 2000

The Clue of Nature's Nitroglycerine

You know that one way to dilate or open a dangerously tight coronary blood vessel emergently is with nitroglycerine. Well, why wait for an emergency? We need more healing nutrients and oxygen delivered to our cells all the time. Luckily we make our own vasodilating nitroglycerine. We make nitric oxide in the walls of our blood vessels. **We make our own "nitro", called nitric oxide, out of an amino acid from our foods, called arginine**. So I guess it might not surprise you to learn that if humans are given extra of this amino acid (that we can't live without), they promote relaxation in their blood vessels and the blood pressure goes down, all without drugs.

The dose varies with the individual and how many other abnormalities he has to fix. But it is safe to use anywhere from 500 to 6000 mg twice a day. It comes as a lower dose sustained release form, **Perfusia** or the pure powder, **Arginine Powder** for greater doses and ease. And **arginine makes the body take-up more magnesium** (Dai), while **correcting magnesium can also help correct potassium**, another mineral wasted by diuretics (Rude). For example, often when a person is prescribed a diuretic, the potassium goes down. Try as he might with prescription potassium, the cardiologist finds it won't correct, and neither will the arrhythmia or weakness. Giving **magnesium beautifully corrects recalcitrant potassium deficiency**. So it's another win-win situation when you take nutrients, for they harmonize in concert.

Evidence:
• Rude RK, Physiology of magnesium metabolism and the important role of magnesium in potassium deficiency, *Am J Cardiol,* 63:31G-34G, 1989
• Dai L-J, et al, Glucagon and arginine vasopressin stimulate Mg2+ uptake in mouse distal convoluted tubule cells, *Am J Physiol*, 274:F328-F335, 1998
• Bonnet S, et al, A mitochondria-K+ channel axis is suppressed in cancer and its normalization promotes apoptosis and inhibits cancer growth, *Cancer Cell*, 11:37-51, 2007

The Mystery of How the Sick Get Sicker, Quicker

Now some folks have a glitch in their chemistry; they make an enzyme that kills this arginine that directs vasodilatation chemistry. But it can be easily fixed once you know it is there. A simple test, the **ADMA,** diagnoses this. Oddly, most cardiologists never heard of it. That is because the focus with blood tests in medicine is to see if we need another drug, not to determine what nutrients are needed for repair. And nutrients are the only thing that will repair or fix this ADMA-caused arginine deficiency.

Lots of other categories of drugs are used for hypertension, like a family of drugs called **beta-blockers** (you can usually tell these because their names often end in –ol, like atenolol). These **deplete zinc, raise triglycerides, usher in diabetes, lower the protective HDL cholesterol, and poison your thyroid hormone** so that it actually cannot convert T4 to its active form, T3 (Kayser). You get the picture. Every drug has a list of bad side effects plus nutrients it steals from the body as well, making sure you will get sicker, and need more drugs. And the **guidelines for medicine do not include testing for these created deficiencies**.

Evidence:
- Kayser L, et al, The thyroid function and size in healthy men during three weeks treatment with beta-adrenergic antagonist, *Horm Metab Res*, 23:35-37, 1991

The Clue of the Vitamin D Debacle

Another category of drugs used commonly for high blood pressure is ACE inhibitors (<u>a</u>ngiotensin <u>c</u>onverting <u>e</u>nzyme inhibitors, Lisinopril® as an example, etc.), meaning they poison this enzyme in the kidney, thus bringing the pressure down. Wouldn't it be great if there were a natural nutrient that could take the place of poisoning the kidney enzyme? There is. It is vitamin D.

The only problem is there is a hidden epidemic of vitamin D deficiency in the U.S. If that were not enough, the amount recommended is far too low and archaic. Leading specialists around the world have proven it should no longer be 400 I.U. a day, but more like 2000-4000 I.U. And to make matters worse, foods and milks fortified with vitamin D2 use the cheap synthetic form that counters many of the good effects of real vitamin D3. What determines this old fashioned low dose is that we no longer get rickets. But vitamin D does a lot more than prevent that.

Merely fixing the level of **vitamin D can accomplish the same thing as an ACE inhibitor** for many folks, and with a lot better health benefits thrown into the package. For example, healthy levels of vitamin D are also needed to keep folks from diabetes, depression, multiple sclerosis, osteoporosis, leg weakness, tooth loss, falls and accidents, and cancer, as well as arteriosclerosis. In fact just having **a low "normal" vitamin D level can double your risk of heart disease.** That makes a vitamin D deficiency more of a risk factor than some forms of high blood pressure.

In fact, your chance from dying from any heart disease as well as any other seemingly unrelated disease is closely tied to your vitamin D level (Dobnig). But there is a hidden epidemic of vitamin D deficiency. Sadly, the science, even from Harvard School of Public Health, clearly shows that the amount we need in a day is not 400 but 4000 I.U. **Solar D Gems 2000** IU, 1 or 2 a day may be what you need. Of course, *your doctor does not have to work blindly.* He can assay your vitamin D level. Just be sure you see the result and that it falls **way above 100 nmol/L or 40 ng/mL, in fact over 60 ng/ml is preferable** (and don't use the antiquated "norm" found on most lab reports.

Evidence:
• Bischoff-Ferrari HA, et al, Estimation of optimal serum concentrations of 25-hydroxyvitamin D for multiple health outcomes, *Am J Clin Nutr,* 84:18-28, 2006

• Pfeifer M, et al, Effects of a short-term vitamin D(3) and calcium supplementation on blood pressure and parathyroid hormone levels, in elderly women, *J Clin Endocrinol Metab*, 86:1633-7, 2001
• Lind L, et al, Hypertension in primary hyperparathyroidism - reduction of blood pressure by long-term treatment with vitamin D (alphacalcidol). A double-blind, placebo-controlled study, *Am J Hypertens,* (4 Pt I): 397-402, 1988
• Holick MF, Vitamin D: importance in the prevention of cancers, type I diabetes, heart disease, and osteoporosis, *Am J Clin Nutr,* 79; 3:362-71, 2005
• Holick MF, High prevalence of vitamin D inadequacy and implications for health, *Mayo Clin Proc,* 81; 3:353-73, Mar 2006
• Li YC, et al, 1,25-Dihydroxyvitamin D(3) is a negative endocrine regulator of the rennin-angiotensin system, *J Clin Invest*, 110:229-38, 2002

Pain Medication Clue

Among the oodles of reasons one in four people get high blood pressure is that it is a common side effect of very common drugs. For example, **NSAIDs** is short for non-steroidal anti-inflammatory drugs. That includes everything from aspirin and Motrin® (ibuprofen) to the prescription forms (like Celebrex®, Voltaren®, Arthrotec®, Naprosyn®, Clinoril®, Tolectin®, etc. and the withdrawn Vioxx®, which may have quadrupled the heart attack rate). Most medicine cabinets or gym bags contain some form of **this drug category that has a new onset of hypertension as a side effect** (Fitzgerald).

Evidence:
• Fitzgerald GA, Coxibs and cardiovascular disease, *New Engl J Med,* 351; 1:1709-11, Oct 21, 2004

The Lead Clue

Another major cause of high blood pressure that pharmacy-focused cardiologists rarely check for is lead toxicity. This heavy metal tanks up in our kidneys throughout a lifetime from numerous unavoidable sources, from auto exhaust and industrial pollution to food additives, and more. When lead reaches a critical level, you can have high blood pressure. Other equally unavoidable environmental metals do the same, like mercury, arsenic, cadmium and aluminum. If you doubt the magnitude of these pollutants, government journals show that we have so poisoned the world with these that **the polar bears in the Arctic have hypothyroidism and osteoporosis from our chemicals**, and the average newborn baby already has measurable levels in his umbilical cord blood.

Meanwhile, no workup for a curable cause of hypertension is complete without a provocation heavy metal test. Of course, we are all so polluted that it makes sense to just get rid of the heavy metals. A simple detoxifying chemical, **DMSA** or **Captomer**® is available non-prescription (all this and more is described in full, including the testing and treatment in *The High Blood Pressure Hoax*).

Getting the heavy metals out of the body can not only lower blood pressure, but is also a great way to reverse the hands of time and **slow down aging**. In fact when you get rid of heavy metals that you have spent a lifetime accumulating, lots of symptoms melt away that you never dreamed of getting rid of, like arthritis, poor memory, anemia, heart or kidney problems, bizarre nerve, chronic pain or bone disorders, and more.

Evidence:
- Ding Y, et al, Lead-induced hypertension, *Environ Res*, 76:107-13, 1998

The Grainy Solution

You are probably as sick as I am of hearing the recommendation for 5 fruits and vegetables a day. Who could eat that much? The reality is that there is another form of **food that has twice the healing or anti-oxidant capacity as fruits and vegetables, and that is whole grains**. Things like brown rice, whole wheat, buckwheat, barley, oats and millet are just a few. In fact in one study of 88 folks with high blood pressure, **3 out of 4 of them dropped**

their blood pressure medications in half just by having 2 small ½ cup servings of whole grains a day. Plus they dropped their cholesterol and sugar levels.

And other studies show you drop your rate of heart attack, cancer and more. In fact whole grains are 50% of the macrobiotic diet, proven to reverse cancers when folks had exhausted all that medicine had to offer, were bed-ridden on oxygen and given 48 hours to live (Rogers, *TW* 2006). My favorite source of mail order organic non-GMO whole grains is **Natural Lifestyle** (1-800-752-2775). For whole grain recipes, see *Macro Mellow*.

Need something incredibly simple? In one study they merely gave folks **4 stalks of celery a day** and successfully lowered their blood pressure. And of course, whole grains and vegetables are a good source of potassium whose deficiency can be the cause of high blood pressure, and which is lowered by the first treatment, diuretics.

Sometimes a high blood pressure cure can be as simple as getting the sugars out of the diet (Preuss, Martinez, Hwang). **High fructose corn sugar, dextrose, and sucrose are all sugars that can trigger high blood pressure**. They are disguised in "health" drinks, sodas, and a multitude of processed foods. If it is not an easy task to stop these sugar addictions, you want to read *No More Heartburn* to determine if you have a gut full of yeast called Candida that can make you mercilessly crave sugars. Or you may want to assay and correct the mineral deficiencies that cause hypoglycemia, like manganese, magnesium, vanadium, chromium and zinc (directions for this and much more in *The High Blood Pressure Hoax*).

Evidence:

• Dobnig H, et al, Independent association of low serum 25-hydroxyvitamin D and 1, 25-dihydroxyvitamin D levels with all-cause and cardiovascular mortality, *Arch Intern Med*, 168; 12:1340-9, 2008

- Preuss HG, Knapka JJ, Antonovych TT, et al, High sucrose diets increase blood pressure of both salt-sensitive and salt-resistant rats, *Am J Hypertens,* 5:585-91, 1992
- Preuss HG, Effects of chromium and guar on sugar-induced hypertension in rats, *Clin Nephrol*, in press
- Martinez FJ, Rizza RA, Romero JC, High fructose feeding elicits insulin resistance, hyperinsulinemia and hypertension in normal mongrel dogs, *Hypertension,* 23:456-3, 1994
- Young JB, Landsberg L, Stimulation of the sympathetic nervous system during sucrose feeding, *Nature,* 269:615-17, 1977
- Hwang ISs, Ho H, Reven GM, et al, Fructose-induced insulin resistance and hypertension in rats, *Hypertension,* 10:512-6, 1987
- Heckbert SR, Longstreth WT, Furberg CD, et al, The association of antihypertensive agents with MRI white matter findings and with modified min-mental state examination in older adults, *J Amer Geriatric Soc,* 1997; 45:1423-1433
- Psaty BM, Heckbert SR, Furberg CD, et al, The risk of myocardial infarction associated with anti-hypertensive drug therapies, *J American Medical Association,* 1995; 274:620-625
- Fitzpatrick AL, Daling JR, Weissfeld JL, et al, Use of calcium-channel blockers and breast carcinoma risk in postmenopausal women, *Cancer,* 1997; 80:1438-47
- Rogers SA, *Total Wellness 2006*, just ask for a free copy of this issue at prestigepublishing.com

Highlights of the Case So Far

In short, the top concerns of aging folks, mainly (1) loss of brain function, as in Alzheimer's, (2) loss of vision, as in macular degeneration (the leading cause of blindness over 50 years of age), (3) loss of life, as in cancer or sudden heart attack, are all potentiated by the very treatments for hypertension.

But we supposedly take blood pressure medications for a longer and better quality of life. "Medical management" is the standard of care directed by "practice guidelines" (dictated by physicians who may also financially benefit from the pharmaceutical industry while ignoring the knowledge we have that enables us to find the cause, fix it and cure the hypertension, once and for all.

Interrogating the Suspect:
Questions to Ask Your Cardiologist
To Determine if He is Slowly Killing You

Interrogate or even, cross-examine your cardiologist? Unthinkable. Yet **your life rests in his hands, or actually in his brain.** Is he sufficiently trained in molecular cardiology to assay and correct the causes of your hypertension? Many folks use more care in selecting a new auto, cell phone, or stereo system than they do a physician, oftentimes because they do not have the knowledge to select a physician. But if the stereo dies, who cares? If you die, it's a different story.

There are so many ways to lower and permanently CURE high blood pressure that it boggles the mind why we insist on merely bludgeoning it for the rest of our lives with drugs. Especially drugs that guarantee you will require more drugs, while bringing on an avalanche of more side effects, symptoms and diseases. I have given you just a glimpse of how you may be being cheated out of finding the cure for your blood pressure. For all the details and references, read *The High Blood Pressure Hoax.*

For the 10-page comprehensive blood test that includes all the items discussed like your RBC magnesium and RBC potassium, arginine, homocysteine, vitamin D, an unprovoked heavy metal screen, RBC zinc, HDL, and much more, have him order the **Cardio/ION**. These are NOT in the standard chemical profile that all docs do. In fact your cardiologist may have never heard of this test. In the meantime, you want to **test your doctor to determine whether he will be helping or hurting you.** Ask any of the following:

- What tests will you be doing to find the curable causes of my blood pressure?
- What form of magnesium will you be testing?

- Will you be checking my fatty acids? Intracellular potassium? ADMA?
- Will you be doing a heavy metal provocation?
- Would you be willing to give me a trial prescription for the most potent form of magnesium?
- What medication are you starting with? Do you think I suffer from a deficiency of this drug?
- What nutrient fixes the problem without a drug?
- Will you be checking my homocysteine level?
- What further tests will you do if the first attempts don't find the cause, so I don't need a lifetime sentencing on some drug?
- Are you willing to read a concise book by a physician with all the evidence and instructions for the sake of my health and to expand your knowledge?

Solution Sources

Item	Web/Company	800#
Cardio/ION, ADMA	metametrix.com	221-4640
Natural Lifestyle	natural-lifestyle.com	752-2775
Cod Liver Oil, E Gems Elite	carlsonlabs.com	323-4141
Chelated Magnesium	carlsonlabs.com	323-4141
Arginine Powder	carlsonlabs.com	323-4141
Solar D Gems 2000	carlsonlabs.com	323-4141
PhosChol	nutrasal.com	777-1886
Natural Calm	supervites.net	888-800-1180
Magnesium Chloride Solution	windhampharmacy.com	518-734-3033
DMSA	vrp.com	877-2447
Captomer, Perfusia	needs.com	634-1380
The High Blood Pressure Hoax	prestigepublishing.com	846-6687

Chapter II

The Mistaken Case of High Cholesterol

If you think folks with high blood pressure get cheated out of finding a permanent cure, the cholesterol problem is even worse. In a nutshell, **cholesterol is not the villain, merely the messenger**. The number one category of cholesterol-lowering drugs is called statins. Lipitor® is the leading seller, in fact the highest grossing drug in the history of the world, grossing over $13 billion last year. No, that is not a typo. It is not million, but billion, over five times the annual budget of the whole FDA.

Statins, a Cruel Crime Perpetrated On the Body

For starters, statins are one of the most dangerous drugs ever made. **You don't poison the liver's ability to make cholesterol and get away with it, at least not alive**. You see, you must have cholesterol to make your hormones, like testosterone for libido, thyroid for energy and weight control, and adrenal stress hormone. Cholesterol is needed not only by all your glands, but all your glands are needed to keep you from a heart attack. In a nutshell, cholesterol is the primary ingredient in all your cell membranes, and the starter molecule for most hormones. Without continual repair and replenishment, you get disease and die. Since the cell membrane is like the computer keyboard of the body, all the messages for the body's functions emanate from here.

If that were not important enough, there is a kidney bean-shaped little organ inside of our cells where God's miracle of creating energy from food molecules (that means the difference between life and death) occurs. This bean-shaped microscopic energy factory inside our cells, called *mitochondria*, is full of membranes looped back and forth over one another. It has a **heavy requirement for cholesterol, or the electricity that creates the body's energy just doesn't exist**. Folks end up with chronic diseases like fatigue, depression, fibromyalgia and heart disease. We also need cholesterol for bile for digestion, detoxification and fighting bugs in the gut, to make the happy hormones in the brain for contentment and happy mood, and much more.

So if you poison such basic chemistry as cholesterol, you guessed it. You are in for some serious side effects and rapid aging. So it may not surprise you that thousands of folks have allegedly died from these drugs. The side effects range from aches and pains and bizarre tendon ruptures to provoking lethal heart failure, serious amnesia without warning, Alzheimer's, increased cancer rate, and the ushering in of many other diseases. How does this one category of drugs do so much damage?

It turns out that **the same liver enzyme (HMG CoA reductase) that is poisoned by statins is also needed to make other important things, like our vitamin-like substance coenzyme Q10 or CoQ10** for short. When you don't make enough of this, and/or poison CoQ10 synthesis you can get congestive heart failure for one. This is more serious than cancer because you die sooner and more folks die of it than cancer each year (more on that in the congestive heart failure chapter). Anyone on a statin should take daily coenzyme Q10, as numerous studies prove it reduces your chances of the potentially fatal side effects of the drug (Young). Since we have enough nutrients to take by mouth, I love those dissolved under the tongue, sublingually, whenever I can find them. We have checked this one out for great absorption via blood tests. Dissolve 2-3 **Q-ODT** ("oral dissolving tablet") under your tongue 2-3 times a day.

And as with other nutrients that are depleted by drugs, CoQ10 shares this in common with them. Their initial deficiencies, even before the drug was started, may be the underlying hidden cause of the malady in the first place. In other words, **for some folks, correcting CoQ10 can correct their high cholesterol.** But when you bludgeon the cholesterol with a drug that also lowers the CoQ10, you can get worsening; a cholesterol that won't budge with meds, an eventual rise in cholesterol in spite of medications, or an arm's length of side effects that are seemingly unrelated. For CoQ10, like other nutrients, works in concert with body chemistry to control all disease.

Evidence:
- Folkers K, et al, Lovastatin decreases coenzyme levels in humans, *Proc Natl Acad Sci USA*, 87:8931-4, 1990
- Young JM, et al, Effect of coenzyme Q10 on myopathic symptoms in patients treated with statins, *Am J Cardiol*, 99; 10:1409-12, 2007

There is More to This Crime

But the damage doesn't stop there. **Statins lower your zinc,** which in turn creates a wide range of problems, depending on which of your over 200 zinc-dependent enzymes are affected. If it is the enzyme that changes vitamin B6 into a useable form (pyridoxine kinase) that suffers from lack of zinc, then you get early heart disease, Alzheimer's, blindness from macular degeneration, and/or depression for starters. Or if it affects the enzyme that repairs your genetics (DNA polymerase), then you get gene damage that leads to auto-immune disease like rheumatoid arthritis or MS, or you get cancer. Now mind you we only talked about 2 of the over 200 zinc enzymes' functions.

But let's see what else the statin cholesterol-lowering drugs deplete. Selenium is lost, a priceless mineral whose deficiency leads to prostate or thyroid problems, cancer and inability to detoxify the daily load of chemicals that hasten disease and aging. In some men with enlarged prostates, **just correcting low selenium can bring their PSA back to normal** (evidence in *TW 2008; TW = Total Wellness*, my monthly referenced newsletter of 20 years).

Statins also deplete vitamin E, a vitamin proven in scores of studies to cut your risk of dying of heart disease in half. Now if you were suckered into believing the hype on TV in the past years denigrating vitamin E's effectiveness, you need to know why it came out looking so bad. They didn't use real vitamin E, which contains 4 tocopherols and 4 tocotrienols. I know I promised to make this simple and free from tough science, but it boggles my mind how they could be so stupid and that is being kind. If you only use one part of the **eight parts of vitamin E**, of course it won't work. It wasn't designed that way. It would be *like buying only one out of every eight parts of a car and expecting it to run.* The more serious fact is that most folks are already deficient in vitamin E. For example, a study of kids ages 1-5 from wealthy families in the U.S. showed that 95%, nearly all of them, were already deficient in vitamin E. And no one knows it, because few pediatricians check this crucial nutrient that has been slowly processed out of our diets.

Statins do a lot more damage, but I think you get the point that they not only guarantee worse heart disease, but cancer and brain rot. So why did your cardiologist prescribe a statin for you? Because of a study that showed statins cut your chance of dying of a heart attack by 26%. Wow! Now you see why they even recommend them for folks who do not even have high cholesterol. So where is the problem? In the details.

It turns out that even though the death rate from heart attacks was cut by 26%, the **overall survival was a wash with statins because there were 26% more deaths from accidents, suicides, cancers** and other causes. But the researchers conveniently left this fact (that the overall mortality was unchanged) out of the quickie summary and out of the news reports. So if your doc recommends statins for this reason, he did not read the actual paper and gets his information that your life depends on from the drug detail man/woman, newspapers and TV, just like you do. You need to do better.

Evidence:

- Newman TB, Hulley SS, Carcinogenicity of lipid-lowering drugs, *Journal of the American Medical Association*, 275; 1:555-60, 1996
- Engelberg H, Low serum cholesterol and suicide, *Lancet,* 229; 8795:727-9, 1992
- Meske V, et al, Blockade of HMG-CoA reductase activity causes changes in micro-tubule-stabilizing protein tau via suppression of geranylgeranylpyro-phosphate formation: implications for Alzheimer's disease, *Europ J Neurosci*, 17:93102, 2003

Innocent Reparations:
Lowering Cholesterol Safely is Easy

You would be amazed at how many non-prescription ways there are to lower your cholesterol, and without the vicious harm that statins wield. **Niacin-Time** works better than the prescription drug Niaspan®, while **Policosanol** can work more safely than statins. As well, magnesium acts like a statin in controlling cholesterol, while giving only good side effects that you learned about in the preceding chapter. And vitamin E lowers cholesterol, but only if you use all 8 parts, as in 1-2 **E Gems Elite** and 2 **Tocotrienols** each twice a day and one **Gamma Tocopherol**.

The side effects from **all 8 parts of natural vitamin E** (not some synthetic molecule made in a lab that acts like a monkey wrench in your chemistry)? It repairs the lost vitamin E in cell membranes and **can even make coronary plaque melt away**. And it **reduced the heart attack rate not 26% like statins touted, but better by 33%** while boosting so many other good things like fighting cancers, aging (measured by a blood test called lipid peroxides), and more. Plus real **vitamin E works better than aspirin** and without **doubling your risk of stroke and intestinal hemorrhage like aspirin does**. You should fire your cardiologist if he recommends aspirins, since many nutrients work better, and the scientific evidence, of course, supports this (evidence for every statement in this chapter is in *The Cholesterol Hoax).*

The Wrong Suspect Has Been Incriminated:
Cholesterol Isn't the Bad Guy

The saddest thing about the cholesterol hype is that there are other parameters that are **four times more predictive of early heart attacks than is cholesterol**. So why doesn't your cardiologist do them? Perhaps because Lipitor® is an over $13 billion a year blockbuster drug and the other parameters are fixed easily with far less expensive, non-patented nutrients. There is generally less money to be made from nutrients. **If your cardiologist has prescribed Lipitor® and has not checked your homocysteine, hs CRP, fibrinogen, insulin, lipid peroxides, vitamin E including gamma tocopherol, vitamins D and K, and more, then you have been clearly cheated.** I would fire him if he cannot improve.

These tests are what I call crystal ball tests, because they are more powerful indicators of early death than cholesterol (Ridker). In fact, did you know that **half the folks who have a heart attack never even had high cholesterol** (Ridker)? Cholesterol is not the demon it has been made out to be. It is merely a messenger shouting that the fires of inflammation are raging and the cause should be found and repaired before a heart attack occurs. In the meantime, cholesterol comes to the rescue and acts like a band-aid patching up the holes that free radicals (from environmental chemicals and nutrient deficiencies) have drilled in cell membranes. This is how it contributes to ushering in disease.

Evidence:
* Ridker PM, Hennekens CH, Buring JE, Rifai N, C-Reactive protein and other markers of inflammation in the prediction of cardiovascular disease in women, *N Engl J Med,* 342:836-43, 2000

Solving the Mystery of How Heartburn
Can Lead to a Heart Attack

There is a very common bug, H. pylori (*Helicobacter pylori*), that is in 2 out of 3 folks' stomachs. It can live there with no symptoms, or cause heartburn, GERD (**g**astro**e**sophageal **r**eflux **d**isease), ulcers, stomach cancer, or rot out the stomach lining (called atrophic gastritis) and accelerate aging by stopping absorption of B12 or assimilation of other nutrients. Or **this common stomach bug can migrate to the coronary arteries and drill holes in them, forcing cholesterol to come along to literally patch things up**. But if your cardiologist doesn't test for it, how will he get rid of it? (See *No More Heartburn* for the diagnosis and treatment.) There are other common bugs to be tested for as well, like *Chlamydia pneumoniae*, since its antibodies are found in 79% of arteries that have plaque versus only 4% of normal arteries (details for diagnosis and cure in *The Cholesterol Hoax*).

Nix on Nexium®-Prescribers

By the way, another **simple test of a non-thinking doc** whom you should fire is whether he prescribes Nexium®. You see Prilosec® was the first "blockbuster" drug in the history of the world, in fact the term originated with it. But when its patent expired, it became very cheap. It went from over $3 per capsule to around 30 cents. In order to make a "new" drug that could have a patent which includes exclusive rights to make and charge inflated prices again, researchers merely added a little side arm onto the old Prilosec® molecule. Now it qualified as a new drug, named Nexium®. But in order for it to work in the body, you first have to metabolize the side arm chain **off** the Nexium®. This leaves you with Prilosec®.

The astounding difference is not only that Nexium® is over $3 a capsule and Prilosec® is less than 30 cents. In order to take the side arm off Nexium®, your body uses up precious vitamins, minerals, amino acids, and fatty acids that should have been used for healing and protecting you from premature aging and cancer. So **what self-respecting physician would prescribe something that is more than 10 times more expensive and drains your body of nutrients?** Only someone who does not have an inkling of what it is and how it works. He has no idea of the chemistry of the drug he is licensed to prescribe. You might also find it interesting to know that once Prilosec® came off patent and became generic, it also magically no longer required a prescription and was deemed safer for you, available over-the-counter. How do you think that happened? (By the way, to fix your intestinal problem so you don't need Nexium®; read *No More Heartburn*).

Forensic Clues Find the Cause

So now you know a few of the non-prescription items that can bring your cholesterol to normal. But the smarter of you will want to **discover why it was up in the first place; for it is a messenger that is screaming that inflammation is raging.** You want to find the cause and get rid of it once and for all. Also you want to see if you have any of the **other warning signs that are far more serious than high cholesterol**. You can get much of this accomplished with the **Cardio/ION** blood and urine test. If you have trouble getting it ordered, consult the instructions in *The Cholesterol Hoax*. And in there you will learn about all the causes from hidden bugs, food contaminants, environmental chemicals, heavy metals, and much more.

The beauty of it all is that once you cure your high cholesterol, you have also made a huge step in your anti-aging program for the rest of your life. For if you had not found the cause and gotten rid of it, and merely bludgeoned your system with a statin, you would eventually succumb to not only the side effects of the drug, but of not having discovered the curable causes and letting the situation worsen. Are you willing to experience an avalanche of new symptoms? If you cannot afford to do the blood test, the book also spells out the most commonly low nutrients to take plus their doses, brands, and sources. High cholesterol is curable, and certainly not worth taking a statin drug that you can die from, or that can usher in sudden amnesia or Alzheimer's.

Bad Counsel:
When Your Doctor Wants You to Take a Drug
To Raise Your HDL

Not all cholesterol is bad. In fact, there is good cholesterol that acts like a wheelbarrow and carts bad cholesterol right to the liver where it is dumped into bile and into the gut to be removed permanently. This HDL (high density lipoprotein) cholesterol has been known for decades. However, like many things in medicine, you didn't hear very much about it, merely because there wasn't a drug for it. But now that pharmaceutical companies finally have drugs to focus on HDL, expect to hear a lot more about the importance of raising your HDL. And to raise HDL is indeed a good thing, since many folks who died of heart disease never had high cholesterol, but they did have a low or even "low normal" HDL (in the 30's and 40's). Meanwhile, the first HDL-raising drug was rapidly removed from the market because of increased deaths, but others have followed.

Your level of HDL is much more important than how much of the bad cholesterol, LDL, you have. HDL is so important that many **people who have had serious cardiac valve replacements and heart attacks never had high cholesterol. They only had an HDL in the <u>normal range</u>, but less than 60** (Morgan). This study also confirms that the current "normal" range for HDL is wrong and it should be well above 60.

Because **HDL is the one form of cholesterol in the body that acts like a wheelbarrow, carrying cholesterol away from the coronary arteries** and dumping it into the bile (where we use it for detoxification of body chemicals), **HDL does double duty. It protects us against coronary artery plaque as well as helps us**

detoxify our daily onslaught of chemicals that trigger heart disease. Of course, many natural nutrients and phytochemicals (parts of foods) help to raise HDL beautifully. In fact the average person couldn't take all the natural things that raise HDL. For example, vitamins C and B3 (**Niacin-Time** that you learned about) raise HDL and minerals like magnesium do, as well as amino acids like taurine and carnitine (Hallfrisch, Handler, Mochizuk, Morgan, Rossi). The detoxifier and precursor to glutathione, N-acetyl cysteine or **NAC** also raises HDL, as do the **Tocotrienols**, part of vitamin E that you also learned about (Franceschini, Qureshi).

And this list of nutrients doesn't even begin to touch the surface. Wouldn't it be wonderful if someone put many of these nutrients into one product? Well they did. It's called **HDL Rx**. Take 1-2 twice a day (Integrative Therapeutics). You can start with two capsules three or four times a day and see if this is sufficient to raise your HDL. The constituents are lower doses than those used in studies to raise HDL, because when you combine the symphony of nutrients you can usually get away with much lower doses of individual components.

And if you need, you can certainly add your **Niacin-Time**, the 3 forms of vitamin E, and extra magnesium that you learned about that are so beneficial (Itoh). Orchestrated natural solutions certainly beat taking a prescription medication whose ingredients don't have all the additional benefits that a proprietary blend of multiple nutrients like **HDL Rx** does. And HDL Rx doesn't have a laundry list of side effects like a drug does.

Evidence:
- Morgan J, et al, High-density lipoproteins subfractions and risk of coronary artery disease, *Curr Atheroscler Rep*, 6; 5:359-65, Sept 2004
- Hallfrisch J, et al, High plasma vitamin C associated with high plasma HDL-and HDL-2 cholesterol, *Am J Clin Nutr,* 60; 1:100-105, July 1994
- Morgan JM, et al, The effects of niacin on lipoproteins subclass distribution, *Prev Cardiol,* 7; 4:182-7, Fall 2004

- Itoh K, et al, The effects of high oral magnesium supplementation on blood pressure, serum lipids,and related variables in apparently healthy Japanese subjects, *Brit J Nutr,* 78:737-50, 1997
- Rossi CS, et al, Effect of carnitine on serum HDL-cholesterol: report of two cases, *Johns Hopkins Med J,* 150; 2:51-4, Feb 1982
- Mochizuki H, et al, Increasing effect of dietary taurine on the serum HDL-cholesterol concentration in rats, *Biosci Biotechnol Biochem,* 62; 3: 578-9, Mar 1998
- Handler SS, Rorvik D, eds, Taurine In: *PDR® for Nutritional Supplements,* Montvale New Jersey, Medical Economics Co, 442-4, 2001
- Franceschini G, et al, Dose-related increase of HDL-cholesterol levels after N-acetylcysteine in man, *Pharmacol Res,* 28; 3:213-18, Oct/Nov 1993
- Qureshi AA, et al, Dose-dependent suppression of serum cholesterol by tocotrienols-rich fraction (TRF 25) of rice bran in hypercholesterolemia, humans, *Atheroscler,* 161; 1:199-207, Mar 2002

Beware of Being Thrown Off the Path

Some cardiologists are really into fine-tuning the types of cholesterol that you have, but then they fall short of their mission by not knowing enough chemistry to repair those pathways. Instead they further bludgeon your lipids with more drugs. For example, it is known that having **a high HDL** (high density lipoprotein) **can override the risk of high cholesterol**. Remember having a high HDL (acts **like a wheelbarrow that carries cholesterol off the coronary artery walls**) is protective of your longevity, even in the presence of high cholesterol. Many people have had serious cardiac valve replacements, stents and bypass surgery as well as lethal heart attacks with no cholesterol problems. Their only abnormality was they had a normal HDL, but it was in the lower range of normal, and below the optimum of 60.

One of the many **nutrients that can boost HDL is DHA** (docosahexaenoic acid), a component of cod liver oil. Unfortunately, if it is not properly balanced with the other part of cod liver oil EPA, that can negate its benefit (Mori). That's why measurement and balancing is very important. For now you might want to add one **Super DHA** daily to your nutrients, since we usually find it low.

Or sometimes cardiologists will measure the size of the bad cholesterol, LDL. Again **DHA changes the LDL to the larger size that is more protective as well as helps lower triglycerides** (Mori), plus it drags the bad LDL out of the liver (Vasandani). On the flip side, the trans fats in french fries, mayonnaise, commercial salad dressings, chips and other processed foods tend to make smaller LDL, the one that promotes heart attacks (Mauger). Yet I see many folks who have had LDL particle size and HDL's measured, but then their cardiologists didn't know what natural supplements to use to repair the abnormalities, so he just gave more statin drugs. And worse, he never taught about the importance of avoiding trans fats.

The Cod Connection

Fixing the cell membrane is often the cure for high cholesterol. Don't forget that cholesterol is like a band-aid, patching up holes in the cell membrane (from destructive free radicals). Once you repair the membrane, the body no longer has to send out incredible amounts of band-aids. And on the flip side, if you are on a statin drug, you are poisoning the ability of your liver to make cholesterol for it's best band-aid. You will really go down the tubes faster as unpredictable tendon ruptures, memory loss, personality decline, bizarre body aches and literally every symptom you can think of can arise. In one study alone of over 11,000 folks who had had a heart attack, giving a teaspoonful of **cod liver oil a day and some vitamin E caused a staggering 45% drop in death rate** (GISSI). No drug does that and certainly statins don't even come close. In fact they make the situation worse by lowering both of these!

If your cardiologist is schooled in pharmaceuticals and unschooled in nutritional medicine, he won't even think of measuring and prescribing the correct dose of omega-3 (EPA and DHA) fatty acids for you. In that case, at least a teaspoon of **Cod Liver Oil** a day and one **Super DHA** covers what a majority of folks we measure are sorely deficient in. The reason you need extra DHA when it is already part of cod liver oil? Most folk's ability to convert more EPA to the amount of DHA as needed to protect the heart by lowering blood pressure, cholesterol, triglycerides arrhythmias, angina and plaque is poisoned by an unavoidably common pollutant you will learn about. And don't forget that **PhosChol** should parallel your dose of Cod Liver Oil here as well (Smaby), for that constitutes the "meat" of the membrane sandwich as well as being another "wheelbarrow" to carry the bad cholesterol away.

If your problem is high triglycerides instead of (or in addition to) high cholesterol, again, cod liver oil is your best correction for starters, and sometimes all you will need. The sad part is this is not new information, and has been known for over 2 decades and new information keeps surfacing (Park, Harris). This is inexcusable, but sadly it's the "norm". **If your cardiologist doesn't know the nutritional molecular biochemistry of your body, he will bludgeon your triglycerides with a side effect-ridden drug and fail to measure and correct your fatty acids.** And don't forget that many categories of drugs the cardiologist prescribes, like B-blockers (names usually end in –ol) actually create high triglycerides, diabetes, low thyroid, zinc depletion, and other heart risk factors that contribute to early heart death.

If you are really new to this type of control over your symptoms, at least eat a can of good quality sardines (in spring water with the whole animal present, not skinless) a day for lunch (on whole wheat toast with tamari, mustard or other condiment if you prefer). But get those omega-3s into you. For as you will learn, they make plaque literally slip off the arterial wall. For more information on cholesterol see *The Cholesterol Hoax.*

Meanwhile, clobbering cholesterol with a statin is for amateurs who know nothing of God's miraculous biochemistry of the human body. Start your oil change with the cod correction.

Evidence:

- Mori TA, et al, Purified eicosapentaenoic and docosahexaenoic acids have differential effects on serum lipids and lipoproteins, LDL particle size, glucose, insulin and mildly hyperlipidemic men, *Am J Clin Nutr*, 71:1085-94, 2000
- Mauger JF, et al, Effect of different forms of dietary hydrogenated fats on LDL particle size, *Am J Clin Nutr*, 78:370-5, 2003
- Vasandani C, et al, Upregulation of hepatic LDL transport by n-3 fatty acids in LDL receptor knockout mice, *J Lipid Res,* 43:772-84, 2002
- Park Y, et al, Omega-three fatty acid supplementation accelerates chylomicron triglyceride clearance, *J Lipid Res,* 44:455-63, 2003
- Harris WS, et al, Reduction of postprandial triglyceridemia in humans by dietary n-3 fatty acids, *J Lipid Res,* 29:1451-60, 1988
- Smaby JM, et al, Phosphatidylcholine acyl unsaturation modulates the decrease in interfacial elasticity induced by cholesterol, *Biophys J,* 73:1492-1505
- Lee KW, et al, The role of omega-3 fatty acids in the secondary prevention of cardiovascular disease, *Q J Med*, 96:465-80, 2003
- GISSI-Prevenzione Investigators, dietary supplement with n-3 polyunsaturated fatty acids and vitamin E after myocardial infarction: results of the GISSI-Prevenzione trial, *Lancet*, 354:447-55, 1999

The Clues Continue to Mount

Even though you don't have high blood pressure, be sure you take the things in that chapter, as well. For example, vitamin D is not only important to lower blood pressure, but to keep coronary arteries from tanking up on calcium and cholesterol (Watson), the very reason you were told to take a statin. And as long as I have been at this, it still boggles my mind how old information like this is from such high profile cardiology journals. Does anybody read anymore? Meanwhile, as any good detective does, you should remember all the clues you get, not only from your current case, but also from previous ones. For this constitutes your store of knowledge and determines how effectively and quickly you solve any case.

I could fill a book (and have, in *The Cholesterol Hoax*) on the dangers of cholesterol-lowering drugs and the many superior natural ways to permanently fix lipid concerns, whether too high, too low, or "just right". But lest you are enticed to take the easy road, because the drug is only once a day and your insurance covers it, let me remind you there are no free rides. One in three men get prostate cancer. One mineral that can make the prostates early warning blood test, the PSA (prostatic specific antigen), go back to normal is selenium. Plus a deficiency of selenium (like CoQ10) is one of the factors that contribute to folks dying from statin-induced rhabdomyelitis. Yet this mineral is silently made deficient by statins (Moosmann). Is it really worth taking the easy road?

Evidence:

- Moosmann B, et al, Selenoprotein synthesis and side-effects of statins, *Lancet*, 363:892-4, 2004
- Watson KE, et al, Active serum vitamin D levels are inversely correlated with coronary calcification, *Circulation*, 96:1755-60, 1997

Always Use the Clues You Got From Previous Cases

Nothing you learn in your investigations is useless when it comes to investigating other situations. Just because you learned that magnesium is crucial in correcting high blood pressure, for example, don't ignore that it's also important in high cholesterol. Make sure you accumulate your knowledge through the cases (even if you don't have that particular disease), because you will find you will be able to solve the mysteries and crimes regarding the disease you do have and want to heal a lot faster.

For example, in some people magnesium is the total cure for their hypercholesterolemia. In others it lowers the LDL, makes plaque melt away, raises the HDL, stops angina or arrhythmia, or acts as a calcium channel blocker. So you can see that **a cardiologist who does not measure bare minimum your RBC magnesium**, much less all the other intracellular minerals and fatty acids plus your CoQ10, **has not planned on curing your hypercholesterolemia, nor has he planned on keeping you from dying from the side effects**. He merely plans on bludgeoning your lipids to death with a statin drug for the rest of your life. The saddest thing is that a lot of this evidence has been known for over two decades.

Evidence:
- Rogers SA, Unrecognized magnesium deficiency masquerades as diverse symptoms: evaluation of an oral magnesium challenge test, *International Clinical Nutrition Reviews*, 11; 3:126-130, July 1991 (And I'm a solo country doc, not a university researcher!)
- Rosanoff A, Comparison of mechanism and functional effects of magnesium and statin pharmaceuticals, *J Am Coll Nutr,* 23; 5: 501S-505S, 2004
- Rasmussen HS, et al, Influence of magnesium substitution therapy on blood lipid composition in patients with ischemic heart disease, *Arch Intern Med,* 149: 1050-53, 1989
- Rayssiguier Y, et al, The effect of magnesium deficiency on lipid metabolism in rats fed a high carbohydrate diet, *J Nutr,* 111: 1876-83, 1981

Interrogating the Suspect:
Questions to Ask Your Cardiologist
To Determine If He Is Slowly Killing You

- What tests are you going to look at along with my cholesterol to determine my heart death risk? (It had better include bare minimum homocysteine, hs CRP, RBC magnesium, EPA, DHA, trans fats (palmitolaidic), fibrinogen, insulin, lipid peroxides, vitamin E including gamma tocopherol.)
- If I do take a statin, what nutrients are you going to check for depletion that stems from the drug? (If he doesn't check RBC zinc, CoQ10, alpha and gamma tocopherols, RBC selenium and folate, he doesn't know statins deplete these and more.)
- Are there any safer ways to naturally lower my cholesterol? (Yes, over half a dozen, and without side effects.)
- What tests are you going to do to find the cause of my high cholesterol? (It should include the Cardio/ION, because it is the only test that looks at all the vitamins, minerals, fatty acids, plus the above risk factors and more, whose deficiencies provide the clues to finding the root causes of disease.)

- What kind of diet do you prescribe? (It should not eliminate your favorite eggs, meats, wine and cheeses, but be free of trans fats and any hydrogenated oils, for they cause high cholesterol and Harvard researchers have warned of it for decades.)
- Will we be looking at heavy metals and other xenobiotics? (Mercury, lead, and other heavy metals are discovered by the provocation test, while the deleterious effects of other pollutants like phthalates, Teflon, and fire retardants may be seen in the Porphyrin test. These are described in *The Cholesterol Hoax* and are unavoidable pollutants in this era and common causes of cholesterol elevation.)
- Will we be looking at any infectious agents like H. pylori or *Chlamydia pneumoniae*? (These, too cause high cholesterol.)
- Will we be looking at the balance of my fatty acids? (This is a major repair focus for all disease.)
- Do you recommend aspirin? (If so, he has no knowledge of the chemistry and science behind this fallacy.)
- Do you prescribe Nexium®? (If so, he doesn't even understand the chemistry of the drugs he is licensed to prescribe.)

All the explanations, tests, cures and scientific back up with over 700 references in *The Cholesterol Hoax* are spelled out for you and the physician of your choice who will read and help you go further to cure your high cholesterol.

Solution Sources

Item	Web/Company	800#
Niacin-Time	carlsonlabs.com	323-4141
Super DHA, Cod Liver Oil	carlsonlabs.com	323-4141
Policosanol	protherainc.com	888-488-2488
E Gems Elite, Tocotrienols	carlsonlabs.com	323-4141
Gamma Tocopherol	carlsonlabs.com	323-4141
HDL Rx	integrativeinc.com	931-1709
Q-ODT	intensivenutrition.com	333-7414
PhosChol	nutrasal.com	777-1886

Evidence:

- Rogers SA, *The Cholesterol Hoax*, prestigepublishing.com, 1-800-846-6687
- Rogers SA, *Total Wellness 1999-2009*, prestigepublishing.com, 1-800-846-6687
- Rogers SA, *Macro Mellow*, prestigepublishing.com, 1-800-846-6687
- Rogers SA, *No More Heartburn*, prestigepublishing.com, 1-800-846-6687

Chapter III

The Case of Incurable Life-Threatening Arrhythmias

The Crime Scene

When your heart is thumping away with a chaotic rhythm it will definitely get your attention. The most common arrhythmia is a simple **PVC or premature ventricular contraction**. You know you've had one of these when it feels like your heart has hiccupped or rolled over for a minute. It can feel like a doubly strong beat followed by a microsecond pause and then everything is normal again. These can be triggered by emotional stress, too much coffee, or even caffeine in common over-the-counter cold medications or colas. PVCs are usually sporadic, but if there are several in a minute they can mature into a much more serious arrhythmia. Plus did you know that even **after a heart attack or heart surgery, the most common reason for death is an arrhythmia.** So the bottom line is always get any irregularity checked out.

Any time the heart is not perfectly regular, in its rhythm and intensity or strength of beating, signifies something is broken and should be immediately fixed. **Atrial fibrillation** is a common arrhythmia where the four chambers of the heart are not beating in synchrony. This is usually due to the atrial chambers beating so fast that it would be impossible for the ventricles to keep up. As a result, not every beat from the atria is transmitted to the ventricles. The result is a very irregular or chaotic heartbeat with no rhyme or rhythm.

Thomas Moore in his documented book, *Deadly Medicine*, clearly showed how one prescription anti-arrhythmia drug (Tambocor®) did such a good job at suppressing abnormal compensatory rhythm that over 50,000 patients died. That's more than the combined U.S. deaths from the Vietnam and Korean wars. But don't think that death by anti-arrhythmia drugs stops with that particular drug.

Multiple studies show that **there is a 2½ times increase in death when anti-arrhythmia drugs are used** (Goldberger). That is quite a steep price to be paid for a regular heartbeat. Especially when it's totally curable.

The problem is that some of the arrhythmia drugs are so good that they send the biochemical message, *"Beat regularly, or don't beat at all".* And that is what happens. **Clearly no arrhythmia is a deficiency of any drug that merely works by poisoning electrical pathways in the heart. You need to find and fix what went wrong.**

At this juncture however, I must warn you that you should never go off your anti-arrhythmia drugs until after you have corrected the deficiencies and been arrhythmia-free. And even then your work has just begun. You need to wean off very slowly by cutting the dose a third every month. That's because when you take an arrhythmia drug that blocks various channels and/or receptors on the heart membrane you can't fool the body. It realizes there hasn't been much action around those channels so it makes more receptors to compensate. So if you go off your drugs quickly you can have twice as much arrhythmia as you did before, because you have twice as many receptors. By weaning off slowly you allow those extra compensatory receptors to drop off and the heart to return to normal (further instructions in *The High Blood Pressure Hoax*). Never under-estimate the power of drugs to create "use dependence" (Katz). Make sure to discuss your actions with your doctor.

Evidence:
- Moore TJ, *Deadly Medicine*, Simon and Schuster, New York, 1995
- Goldberger JJ, Treatment and prevention of sudden cardiac death, *Arch Intern Med*, 159:1287, 1999
- Katz AM, Selectivity and toxicity of anti-arrhythmic drugs: molecular interactions with ion channels, *Am J Med,* 104:179-195, 1998

The Detective Work Begins

So why are anti-arrhythmia drugs so dangerous? Because most of the time the underlying cause has not been sought, so the arrhythmia can only worsen. Meanwhile, many researchers have shown what we have witnessed for decades. **You can completely cure atrial fibrillation, PVCs, tachycardia, and other arrhythmias**. It just involves a little detective work. One of the most common things to turn around arrhythmias is magnesium. Yes, as little as 600 mg of magnesium twice a day has totally turned off some people's atrial fibrillation, although the official RDA is only 240-420, depending on year and institution (Eisenberg). In fact, **magnesium deficiency is probably one of the most common causes of atrial fibrillation and other arrhythmias.** I know it was for me when I had ventricular tachycardia, which literally dropped me to the floor unconscious.

Why is there so much arrhythmia? The average diet provides far less than 30% of the amount of magnesium that people need in a day, so most folks are deficient (Nielsen). Furthermore, sweating from sports and saunas, high sugar or processed foods diets, worry, unbalanced high calcium intake, prescription medications, alcohols and more foster magnesium deficiency even faster. The sad part is that some of the studies are fraught with errors.

For one study, they relied on the antiquated RDA (recommended daily allowance) that then was merely 290 mg/day. Since the average person gets a third of the RDA, this means that patients were on less than 100 mg (equals 412 mmol for Europeans) of magnesium a day. The researchers in the study only gave 200 mg additional magnesium to turn around arrhythmias. Obviously it was not sufficient for all the patients, for in 39 years of medical practice I've seen folks who need over 3000 mg of magnesium a day to stop muscle spasms, cramps, high blood pressure, migraines, or arrhythmias. These folks can turn their symptoms on and off like a switch by getting their particular dose. Magnesium deficiency has been a known cause of arrhythmias for over a quarter century (Reyes), so there's really no excuse for ignorance.

Why do some folks need so much magnesium? Many reasons, including the unavoidable environmental heavy metals like **lead and cadmium that damage the mechanism in the kidney to save magnesium**. These folks need more than the average person until their magnesium-losing nephropathy is diagnosed and cured. For the average person the dose sufficient to turn off arrhythmias is around 1000 mg a day, equivalent to ½ teaspoon twice a day of the best form, prescription **Magnesium Chloride Solution**, 200 mg/cc (full prescribing directions in *The Cholesterol Hoax*). If you cannot get a prescription fast enough, start with the non-prescription next best form **Natural Calm** (1-888-800-1180). With 615 mg of magnesium citrate per tablespoon, a heaping teaspoon 2 or 3 times a day will often do the trick. If it creates too much loose stool, refer to *The Cholesterol Hoax* for more details. As well, the citrate helps to alkalinize the urine, thus tending to ward of infections (Spooner), another benefit, plus as a powder you avoid another capsule and it works more quickly.

The prescription form, **Magnesium Chloride Solution**, 200 mg/cc, is so potent it can act like an IV. In fact I have seen it rescue folks from angina, migraines or muscle spasms that pinned them to the floor just by slipping a swig under the tongue and letting it get absorbed like sublingual nitroglycerine. **Mag Chlor 85** is a non-prescription form with 85 mg/ml (versus 200 for the Rx form). So 5 ml equals a teaspoon and gives 420 mg of magnesium for emergencies for folks who can't get the Rx or want a liquid form other than the capsules or the more rapidly absorbed powder.

Evidence:
- Reyes AJ, Pathogenesis of arrhythmogenic changes due to magnesium depletion, *S A Med J*, 311-12, 1983
- Eisenberg MJ, Magnesium deficiency and sudden death, *Am Heart J*, 124; 2:544-49, 1992

- Spooner JB, Alkalinisation in the management of cystitis, *J Int Med Res*, 12:30-34, 1984

The Verdict on the Magnesium Scam

Clearly to treat arrhythmia without checking magnesium is unthinkable to me in view of the overwhelming evidence I've presented in over a dozen books. So why is it ignored? I can find no rationale. Here are some additional facts. In one study of patients admitted to the intensive care unit who were given intravenous magnesium over 10 minutes, the magnesium turned off arrhythmias in seven out of eight patients in those who had an abnormal serum magnesium and in one out of six patients in whom the serum magnesium was normal (of course, they most assuredly had other unidentified deficiencies that accompanied it).

In the group of folks with abnormal serum magnesium, remember these patients had already **failed to have their arrhythmias respond to conventional anti-arrhythmia drugs. That means the docs resorted to drugs without ever having checked the magnesium!** The conclusion or verdict of the clinicians who wrote the paper was that since intravenous magnesium is inexpensive, easy to the give, and has very few side effects, it **should be the therapy of choice in the management of cardiac arrhythmias** (Kasaoka).

But still these researchers did not recommend checking the best and most sensitive test that you learned about, the RBC (red blood cell or erythrocyte) or intracellular magnesium. And they didn't know enough to caution docs against using the notoriously inadequate serum magnesium. In fact, that is what they used in the study. Why is this important? (1) Because less than 1% of magnesium in the body is in the serum. It's like the old joke of the drunk looking for his lost keys under the street lamp because that's where the best light was. In fact the **RBC is 9 times more sensitive an indicator of low magnesium than the serum** (Purvis)!

(2) But a more dangerous reason exists. **As the RBC magnesium goes silently lower inside the cell** where it regulates heart rhythm, **the body compensates by making the serum magnesium higher!** (Nielsen). The result? The unknowledgeable cardiologist who just checks your serum magnesium and finds it normal will be even more convinced he is right in ignoring it. Meanwhile, you **won't be the first patient to go to his deathbed with his cardiologist believing he was right in ignoring correcting magnesium**.

Scores more studies have proven **magnesium is just one of the many minerals that are crucial to control or correct arrhythmias** (Klevay, Feyertag). In fact when you look at all the data, it looks like it should border on malpractice to fail to check an RBC magnesium in every disease, since it underlies not only arrhythmias, but is a major cause of sudden cardiac arrest, heart attacks, heart failure, high blood pressure, high cholesterol, cardiomyopathy, as well as diabetes, Syndrome X (Metabolic Syndrome), osteoporosis, depression, fatigue, muscle spasms mimicking ruptured discs, constipation, and more. I can't imagine why any doctor would prefer to practice blindly and not know the status of the minerals, beginning with magnesium. There are **many other minerals that also contribute to cardiac arrhythmia such as copper, chromium, manganese, zinc, selenium** and more. These are all measurable and the complete details on how to do it and what to take to correct them are in *The Cholesterol Hoax.*

And if the arrhythmia is due to another mineral deficiency like potassium, recall that this is also lowered by diuretics (fluid pills). Unfortunately, sometimes the potassium won't correct, and refractory hypocalemia is diagnosed. That occurs because in many cases **potassium will not correct until the magnesium is first corrected**. Instead unknowledgeable cardiologists keep raising the dose of potassium, which in itself can create cardiac arrhythmias. Clearly if the cardiologist is not measuring RBC magnesium and all the complementary minerals, he has no knowledge of what all the levels are. It is an important balancing act. The patient can die, as many have.

That is what happened in one study published in none other than the *Journal of the American Medical Association*. They proved in a famous Boston hospital that over 54% of patients were low in magnesium (you guessed it, they, too used the inferior serum magnesium, which is why the statistic is so low). The saddest part of the study was that 95% of the doctors taking care of these 1033 patients never ordered even one magnesium lab test all the time these folks were sick enough to be hospitalized (Whang). And of course, many of them died, never to know their arrhythmia or sudden cardiac arrest might have been cured with pennies of magnesium. Did their cardiologists unknowingly contribute to their deaths?

Evidence:
- Nielsen FH, et al, Dietary **magnesium deficiency induces heart rhythm changes**, impaired glucose tolerance, and decreases serum cholesterol in post menopausal women, *J Am Coll Nutr,* 26;12: 121-32, 2007
- Whang R, Ryder KW, Frequency of hypomagnesemia and hypermagnesemia, requested versus routine, *J Amer Med Assoc,* 2634; 3063-4, 1990
- Feyertag J, et al, Effect of low dose oral magnesium supplementation of different magnesium parameters and on ventricular arrhythmias. In Smetana R (ed): *Advances in Magnesium Research: Magnesium in Cardiology: Proceedings of the 5th European Congress on Magnesium"*, London: John Libbey & Company, pp71-77, 1997
- Klevay L, et al, Low dietary magnesium increases supraventricular ectopy, *Am J Clin Nutr,* 75:550-54, 2002
- Purvis JR, et al, Magnesium disorders and cardiovascular diseases, *Clin Cardiol,* 15; 8:556-68, Aug 1992
- Eisenberg MJ, Magnesium deficiency and cardiac arrhythmias, *NY State J Med*, 86; 3:133-6, March 1986

Magnesium is Superior to Drugs

In a study of 57 patients with 3 kinds of arrhythmias, supraventricular tachycardia, atrial fibrillation and atrial flutter, intravenous magnesium was compared with a prescription calcium channel blocker, Verapamil®. Within four hours, over half or 58% of patients receiving magnesium converted to normal (sinus rhythm) and within 24 hours a total of 62% had converted.

So in one day with pennies of magnesium, 2 out of 3 near fatal arrhythmias normalized with one dose of magnesium. But only 1 out of 5 stopped their arrhythmia on the leading drug. Only 19% converted within four hours on Verapamil®. **Magnesium was 300% better in stopping an arrhythmia than a leading cardiology drug.** And of course the failures that didn't get magnesium were electrocuted with cardioversion, as were those for whom magnesium wasn't their only deficiency.

No side effects were observed during magnesium infusion whereas six patients receiving the drug developed serious side effects such as dangerously low blood pressure and signs of cardiac failure. Since the conversion to normal rhythm (1) occurred quicker (and time is of the essence because the longer you have an arrhythmia, the higher your chance of sudden death), plus it was (2) without side effects, and (3) less expensive, it certainly appears to be the treatment of choice, as the researchers agreed. What does your cardiologist use? And this study is over 16 years old in a major cardiology journal! And recall that Verapamil® is a calcium channel blocker, the class that causes MRI-proven brain shrinkage and intellectual rot within 5 years.

Evidence:
- Gullestad, Al, et al., The effect of magnesium versus verapamil on supraventricular arrhythmias, *Clinical Cardiology,* 16: 4 29-4 34, 1993

A Test to Find a Competent Cardiologist

Here's a test to see if you have a superlative cardiologist, worthy of your time, money and the control over your life. Naively ask,

"What significance does tricarballyate have to my heart symptoms?" (Pronounced: tri car bal' y ate).

If you get a blank look or answer designed to slough it off as unimportant, you are probably not in the right place. You see, there is an old saying, "All disease begins in the gut". And it happens that we all get a slew of bad bugs in our guts from eating out, antibiotics, processed foods and more. Some of these bugs, as they are living and growing in our guts, make an excessive amount of (measurable) organic acid, **tricarballyate.** Why do you want to know this? Because this organic acid can act like a claw and **grab onto or chelate out any magnesium that passes by**. So you may tank up on magnesium, but you can't get enough absorbed from the gut to correct your arrhythmia and bring your RBC level to the top quintile in the blood test.

And when I say top quintile, you really want to have a magnesium at the very top, or higher, than normal. Why? Because government regulators in order to standardize lab tests, run hundreds of samples from the populous periodically to re-check the norm. As people get less interested in learning about health, eat more fast foods, take more drugs, and tank up on more pollutants in this unprecedented era, the average amount of magnesium in folks drops dramatically. So they end up with more complaints and take more medications. As an example of one nutrient, 2 years ago the norm for magnesium was 40-80 ppm packed cells, and currently is 15-40.

You will find an elevated tricarballyate on your **Cardio/ION**. The best way to fix this is to have your doctor order a **Comprehensive Stool Test** (Doctor's Data) to find out what bug has overgrown and what can kill it. Sometimes something as simple as **Kyolic Liquid**, an exclusive proprietary aged garlic extract, can often kill the bad bugs in a couple of weeks. Then use a blend of probiotics like **Abx Support** to put the good bugs back in the gut. You really can't go wrong with Kyolic Liquid, since it has so many other cardio-protective attributes, like lowering cholesterol, blood pressure, arrhythmia, slowing progression of coronary calcifications, and much more. Chromium (as you will learn, is one mineral that has cured arrhythmias once it was corrected), is commonly low, and its deficiency makes folks crave sweets. That's why I like a combination of the two products in the form of **Kyo-Chrome**, taken as 2-3 twice a day. If you have trouble curing the gut, see the far more complete *No More Heartburn*, and meanwhile, when magnesium won't correct, think gut.

Evidence:

- Schwartz R, yet al, Effect of tricarballyic acid, a nonmetabolizable rumen fermentation product of trans-aconitic acid, on Mg, Ca and Zn utilization of rats, *J Nutr,* 118; 2:183-88, 1988
- Lord RS, Bralley JA, eds, *Laboratory Evaluations for Integrative and Functional Medicine*, 2nd Ed., metametrix.com, 2008

The Clues Are Endless

I'm giving you an example of magnesium again to drive home several life-saving points. (1) It is an extremely common, yet commonly overlooked nutrient deficiency. (2) Most of the time if it is checked, the wrong assay is done, and (3) by using the wrong assay it gives the unknowledgeable cardiologist an erroneous confidence, dangerously unwarranted. And (4), magnesium is crucial for every cardiovascular diagnosis.

But just because it is the most commonly low and therapeutic nutrient, don't think that magnesium is the end of the line. Just about every nutrient has played a role in reversing arrhythmias, it just depends on the individual's needs. For example, in one study of 40 patients having coronary artery bypass surgery, those who had 150 mg of coenzyme Q10 a day for seven days prior to the operation showed lower incidence of ventricular arrhythmias during the recovery (Chello). Because this is too low a dose and too short a term of treatment it makes a study like this even more convincing.

In another study **CoQ10 taken daily caused a dramatic over 25% drop in abnormal heart rhythms** (Fujioka). And don't forget statins for cholesterol dramatically lower CoQ10. Since it is integral in energy control of the heart and many unavoidable everyday pollutants like plasticizers damage its metabolism, I recommend 1- 3 sublingual **Q-ODT** twice a day.

Another clinician found that selenium had a beneficial effect in keeping arrhythmias controlled. This should not be surprising since it is a component of glutathione peroxidase, a free radical scavenging enzyme that protects the heart muscle (Lehr). Since this mineral also has made (1) prostatic PSA tests return to normal, (2) is crucial in detoxification, and (3) in preventing cancers, and (4) much more, and (5) is frequently low in the diet, I recommend a daily supplement, which contains harmonizing minerals, of one **SeaSel.**

In another study, low plasma potassium concentrations were more consistently found in patients with ventricular fibrillation admitted to a coronary care unit (Higham). Unfortunately, many studies focus on solo nutrients because it is easier to look at one at a time. But **nutrients work in concert like members of an orchestra. Nutrients are not a solo act like drugs.** And of course the potassium level is very dependent on whether or not the potassium channels in the cell membrane are healthy (Wang, Bonnet). It appears to me senseless to treat any arrhythmia without assaying not only magnesium, but also the potassium channels and the cell membrane chemistry that houses them. For **if the potassium channels are not repaired** (which can be enormously easy in some) **the arrhythmia may never correct**. Furthermore, the **damaged potassium channels can then go on to cause sudden cardiac death or cancers**.

Or let's look at an extremely common low mineral that is practically never checked by physicians, intracellular chromium. No it's not just used for plating fenders and bumpers on old vehicles, but it has many indispensable roles in the body from controlling diabetes right on down to controlling whether or not you have an arrhythmia. For example, when a cardiologist is reading an EKG the space between two of the squiggles called **QTc interval** is very important, because it's a **powerful predictor of whether or not you will die shortly. Chromium easily corrects this** (Vrtovec), but only if your doctor thinks of assaying it and correcting it! Yet show me a cardiologist who checks your RBC chromium before doing cardioversion, from which you could die.

This is another reason I would take at least 2 **Kyo-Chrome** daily, since you really can't go wrong. It helps regulate diabetes, protect you from stroke, helps regulate your weight and reduce sweet cravings, reduce unwanted intestinal bugs, and much more. For many more minerals that regulate the electricity of the heart see *The Cholesterol Hoax* for a much more complete list and directions of how to take them and where to get them.

Back to these cell membranes, which contain the receptors for all of the minerals and nutrients, plus many more functions. They are like the computer keyboard for the whole cell. As you will learn, the best way to determine what the cell membrane needs is to measure the very chemicals that the cell membrane is made out of, EPA and DHA (as found in cod liver oil). Plus we measure CoQ10 levels, selenium, intracellular potassium and magnesium, chromium, and much more, all in one test. This is especially important *before* procedures like **cardioversion and ablation, because by repairing the membrane chemistry, you may never need these life-threatening procedures.**

Unfortunately cell membranes are also very vulnerable to attack by environmental chemicals plus toxic trans fatty acids that permeate foods (found in unidentified oils like "soy oil" or hydrogenated or partially hydrogenated oils). When pesticides or trans fats or auto exhaust, for example, damage potassium channels, this can lead to hypertension, congestive heart failure or recalcitrant arrhythmias.

With so many dietary and environmental triggers that can damage membrane ion channels, no wonder adding an anti-arrhythmia drug can be lethal (Katz). You don't need one more chemical in an already chemically damaged system. More on the membranes will follow to clarify and enrich your knowledge even further.

Evidence:

- Katz AM, Selectivity and toxicity of anti-arrhythmia drugs: molecular interactions with ion channels, *Am J Med*, 104: 179-195, 1998
- Higham PD, et al, Plasma potassium, serum magnesium and ventricular fibrillation: a prospective study, *Quart J Med*, 86: 609-6 17, 1993
- Chello M, et al, Protection by coenzyme Q10 from myocardial reperfusion injury during coronary artery bypass grafting, *Ann Thoracic Surg*, 58: 14 27-14 32, Nov. 15, 1994
- Lehr D, The possible beneficial effect of **selenium administration in anti-arrhythmic therapy**, *J Am Coll Nutr*, 13; 5: 4 96-4 98, 1994
- Wang Z, Roles of K+ channels in regulating tumor cell proliferation and apoptosis, *Pflugers Arch-Eur J Physiol*, 448:274-86, 2004
- Bonnet S, et al, A mitochondria-K+ channel axis is suppressed in cancer and its normalization promotes apoptosis and inhibits cancer growth, *Cancer Cell*, 11:37-51, Jan 2007
- Vrtovec M, et al, **Chromium supplementation shortens QTc interval** duration in patients with type II diabetes mellitus *Am Heart J*, 149:632-6, 2005
- Fujioka T, et al, Clinical study of cardiac arrhythmias using the 24 hour continuous electrocardiographic recorder (5th report) - **anti-arrhythmia action of coenzyme Q10** in diabetics, *Tohoku J Exp Med*, 141 supple: 453-63, 1983

Is Electrocution of the Victim Warranted?

When drugs fail to control arrhythmias, then cardiologists try to electrocute or shock the heart back into normal rhythm, called cardioversion. But even **cardioversion with a defibrillator has a 50% increased chance of being more successful if magnesium is given first** (McDaniel). On the flip side, you can defibrillate, cardiovert, or electrocute the heart all you want, but if it doesn't have enough magnesium (and other minerals) to allow the electricity to flow or the right fatty acids in the nerve membranes, it amounts to whipping a dead horse.

In fact the professor of medicine at the cardiac care unit at the University of Maryland School of Medicine states, "It is so safe (magnesium) and inexpensive that I can't think of a reason not to give it" (Gottlieb). If you've been prescribed cardioversion without even a magnesium level to identify one of the most common causes of your arrhythmia, and then to compound the travesty they even want to cardiovert you without measuring or at least priming you with protective magnesium prior to electrocuting you, I would jump off that table so fast!

In a study of 15 patients with atrial fibrillation with tachycardia (a rapid ventricular rate over 100 beats per minute), two grams (2000 mg) of magnesium sulfate were given over one minute intravenously followed by one gram every hour for four hours. At five minutes the ventricular rates were decreased 16%, which is comparable to the same control attainable with digoxin in 4 hours (Hayes).

And for certain congenital arrhythmias, like Wolff-Parkinson-White Syndrome, digoxin is contraindicated, plus it has lots of side effects. But intravenous magnesium sulfate given as two grams (equals 2000 mg) over five minutes produced remarkable slowing and control of the rate. And the patients lived. IV **magnesium was far more successful than a drug**. Meanwhile, **most patients whose hearts are subjected to cardioversion, have never had benefit of the assay of nutrients that could cure their arrhythmias**. And cardioversion in an unprepared heart can be lethal.

We've looked at one mineral as an example. But there are dozens of nutrients. And unfortunately nutrient deficiencies are under-recognized and undiagnosed. In one study of **hospitalized patients up to 50% had undiagnosed deficiencies**, and this was not by any means a sophisticated or comprehensive assessment of nutrients, but rather a very unsophisticated screen (Roubenoff).

Evidence:
- Hayes JV, Effect of **magnesium** sulfate on the ventricular rate **control in atrial fibrillation**, *Ann Emergency Med*, 24; 1:61-64, July 1994
- Merrill JJ, et al. Magnesium reversal of digoxin-facilitated ventricular rate during atrial fibrillation in the Wolff-Parkinson-White Syndrome, *Am J Med*, 97: 25-28, July 1994
- Kasaoka S, et al, Effect of intravenous magnesium sulfate on cardiac arrhythmias in critically ill patients with low serum ionized magnesium, *Japanese Circul J*, 60; 11: 871-75, Nov. 1996
- McDaniel, WC, et al, Effects of magnesium sulfate on electrical ventricular defibrillation, *J Electrocardiol*, 31; 2: 1 37-1 43, 1998
- Gottlieb SS, IV magnesium: a cost-effective anti-arrhythmia, *Emerg Med*, 53, May 1994
- Roubenoff R, et al, **Malnutrition among hospitalized patients: Problem of physician awareness**, *Arch Intern Med*, 147:1462-65, 1987

Police Bulletin:
Deadliest Heart Drug, Amiodarone

I'm scared to death by the number of folks who tell me their doctors prescribed amiodarone for their arrhythmias, like atrial fibrillation. This is one of the deadliest drugs in the entire drug book! Folks say they were told the drug was necessary because their arrhythmia was resistant to cardioversion and ablation. That scares me even more, because it shows the cardiologist electrocuted the heart and then actually permanently burned out parts of the heart in desperation. But then I really felt faint when I saw their medical records and not even one cardiologist had ever looked at the chemistry that gets rid of atrial fibrillation and other arrhythmias permanently. And these folks had limited financial resources and had been to several of the leading cardiology clinics in the United States.

Amiodarone (brand name Pacerone®) is one of the most dangerous cardiac drugs in the *PDR* (*Physicians' Drug Reference*, a book in most public libraries that describes most prescription drugs, their chemistry, indications, side effects, etc.). It is so dangerous that it has the highest level of dangerous warnings called a **black box warning**. The warning for this drug basically translates into telling the physician to **make sure he has done everything for the patient that he can before he prescribes it**, because **this drug has a high chance of killing the patient all by itself**. Basically it's also such a strong anti-arrhythmia drug that it virtually commands the heart to "beat regularly or don't beat at all". And that's unfortunately what happens. Plus as you will see, the longer you are on it the higher your chances climb of having a fatal reaction from it. Let me explain some of the mechanisms that promote fatality.

Amiodarone is 37% by weight made out of iodine. This chemical form of iodine inhibits the conversion of your thyroid hormone T4 into the active form T3. So **the drug can make many people hypothyroid.** This low thyroid function now can lead to high cholesterol, fatigue, constipation, depression, and more. Plus the low thyroid can add to further cardiac arrhythmias, which is what you were taking this dangerous drug for in the first place.

On the flipside, other people go the opposite way and get hyperthyroid on it where the thyroid becomes overactive. This also creates new arrhythmias plus high blood pressure, and it can lead to a heart attack. Unfortunately the standard treatment for continuing or new arrhythmias is often to raise the dose of the drug or add other drugs, which further adds to its dangers including the potential to kill you. Or they resort to cardioversion again, trying to electrocute your heart back into normal rhythm with anywhere from 60-600 joules. In the *PDR (Physicians Desk Reference*, the book that describes all of the prescription drugs) it says the physician must measure the thyroid function and he must do it frequently for anyone on the drug. I rarely see this happen. The drug also has triggered thyroid tumors. And remember other heart drugs also poison the thyroid, like B-blockers, also prescribed for arrhythmias.

Lots of other things happen with the drug amiodarone. For example, its metabolites slowly accumulate just like environmental toxins, and they cannot be removed from the body with dialysis. As well, **it has caused fatal rhabdomyolysis** (the heart and other muscles rot, and waste overloads the kidneys) **just like the statin cholesterol-lowering drugs do**. This begins with early warnings of bizarre muscle and joint aches, but can end in death. It can damage the eyes causing optic neuropathy, and 17% of the people get pulmonary hypersensitivity from which one in ten dies. The fact that there's a 20% (1 in 5 patients) dropout rate tells you it's a pretty nasty drug. And many serious symptom side effects go undiagnosed for months like chronic cough that doesn't let up and no one can figure out. Instead the victim gets further tests to rule out asthma versus heart failure, which adds unnecessarily to the body's radiation level, plus time lost with doctor visits and expense lost to pharmaceutical burdens.

There are many other side effects, but the most common is the fact that it just plain doesn't work. A lot of people get worse arrhythmias, heart block, or ventricular fibrillation, which can be fatal in minutes. Why does amiodarone have such a poor track record and why is it so frequently fatal? Because the majority of physicians that prescribe amiodarone don't look for the curable causes of atrial fibrillation. Even in **the *PDR* it says, "Any potassium or magnesium deficiency should be corrected <u>prior to</u> prescribing this drug."** I rarely see even this done when I review records from folks who have been to some of the most prominent cardiologists and heart centers in the U.S.

Once in a while when I review a cardiologist's and cardiovascular surgeon's records to do a consultation, I will see that they did an inappropriately insensitive serum magnesium and potassium, and that was it. Not one other nutrient or risk factor, just the standard cholesterols, etc. Unfortunately this smacks of severe ignorance of the body chemistry, for recall less than 1% of magnesium is in the serum, and it can look fictitiously normal in spite of deficiencies severe enough to cause death. **Relying on serum magnesium** as opposed to an RBC (red blood cell or erythrocyte or intracellular) is a **hallmark of a dangerously under-educated and totally "clueless" cardiologist** who is contributing to the patient's death. The serum magnesium test is blatantly inappropriate. Even the *Washington Manual* **has warned physicians for decades that the serum magnesium is worthless.**

In many issues of the *TW* newsletter and in many of the books, I have given voluminous data from well-respected researchers from around the world, proving time and again that **magnesium has not been properly assayed until the RBC form has been used. You can have a perfectly normal looking serum magnesium and walk out of a doctor's office and drop dead** from sudden cardiac arrest from being extremely magnesium deficient. The serum magnesium is the wrong test, is too insensitive, and is an inferior and a misleading assay, and should be frankly ignored. When someone is even a tad low on the serum magnesium they are in deep trouble. I apologize for the repetition, but it is so overlooked yet pivotal to survival and cure.

Long-term survival is exactly the same whether people have part of the heart muscle destroyed (ablation) or have drug therapy, because no one has fixed the underlying cause (Ozcan). And ablation is done even though it is known that "**ablation of the atrioventricular node does not eliminate atrial fibrillation**" (Ozcan). **Ablation is serious because there's no getting back any part of the heart that has been burned out. It doesn't re-grow**. This should be an absolute last resort. Why does it have such a high failure rate? Cardiologists have failed to assay the nutrients and have failed to repair the heart chemistry. **Nutrient assay is the very first thing they should have done and yet they *never* did it.** Instead they resorted to **permanently burning out and destroying a part of the heart** when it was already in trouble. Would you smash the red light on your car's dashboard warning of low oil, or check and refill the missing oil?

Evidence:
Ozcan C, Jahangir A, Shen WK, et al, Long-term survival after ablation of the atrioventricular node and implantation of a permanent pacemaker in patients with atrial fibrillation, *New Engl J Med*, 344; 14:1043-51, 2001

The Amiodarone Crime

Amiodarone's use causes more problems including serious fatal adverse reactions in up to 22% of patients, plus elevation of liver enzymes, as it overloads the detox pathways. Of course these detoxification pathways, too, can be measured along with the minerals, fatty acids and other assays that would lead to the cure of the arrhythmia. Meanwhile, it was found that amiodarone's liver toxicity was in part due to free radicals attacking (phospholipids in) the cell membranes of the liver. Fortunately, the antioxidant silibinin decreased the toxicity (Vereckei). If you have to be on amiodarone for a while, at least boost your liver detoxification of it with 1-2 **Super Milk Thistle** three times a day, my preferred form, to lessen the chance of you being the one in five who dies.

Another equally important liver saver is lipoic acid. In fact this and silibinin (silymarin) are so potent in rescuing the liver that they are **both the only known agents** to save folks' lives who have mistakenly eaten poisonous mushrooms. Usually folks die within 48 hours of ingestion, in spite of all that medicine can offer in the emergency room. But these two agents alone have caused unrivalled survival. But you don't want a lipoic acid that just says "lipoic acid" or "alpha-lipoic", for these contain 50% of a form not able to be used by the body. The preferred form is **R-Lipoic Acid.** Use 1-3 R-Lipoic Acid three times a day depending on the potency of the drug you are trying to protect your liver against.

Evidence:
Vereckei A, et al, The role of free radicals in the pathogenesis of amiodarone toxicity, *J Cardiol Electrophysiol*, 4; 2: 161-177, Apr 1993

The Vicious Cycle:
One Poison Leads to Another

Remember, all drugs merely work by poisoning a pathway in God's miraculous biochemistry. A drug accomplishes turning off the symptom usually, but at what expense? Eventually the symptoms and subsequent side effects (that invariably arise) dictate the need for yet another poison.

When an arrhythmia is recalcitrant and won't turn off with the first drug, the under-educated physician merely tries to bludgeon the recalcitrant arrhythmia with another drug, usually a **beta-blocker** (drugs whose names often end in "-ol", like Naldolol®, Atenolol®, Toprol®) for starters. But these not only raise your triglycerides and lower B12; they drop your HDL (which is more dangerous than high cholesterol), and poison the thyroid (creating another cause of arrhythmia). And that is just the beginning. They also cause a silent zinc deficiency. Mind you, zinc deficiency is already very common. Low zinc then leads to any symptom you can think of and usually even seems unrelated, like stomach problems, elevated liver enzymes, high homocysteine (which is 4 times more dangerous than high cholesterol), depression, cancers, fatal infections, Alzheimer's, B6 deficiency, and yes, arrhythmias.

More Clues:
Cod for Cardiac Protection

In our books and newsletters I've given you lots of evidence in the past from the government's leading journals of how **diesel and other vehicular and industrial exhausts damage the heart and lead to arrhythmias, and even cause fatal heart attacks**. One of the main heart-damaging mechanisms of traffic exhaust, for example, is that the heavy metals and volatile organic hydrocarbons are quickly absorbed through the lung and into the bloodstream. Once in the coronary arteries (which feed the heart), environmental **chemicals damage the autonomic nervous system and can**

create any arrhythmia imaginable. No amount of drugs can fix the problem. Folks with the most resistant of arrhythmias need to detoxify these chemicals from the heart (as in *Detoxify or Die*) in order to cure themselves.

But what about preventing chemicals from getting into the heart in the first place? A teaspoon a day of **Cod Liver Oil** can help prevent this. In fact there are scores of papers by researchers across the globe showing that simple things like cod liver oil can also **prevent and/or turn off arrhythmias**, if that is the causative deficiency (Jahangiri, Harris). They have such a good track record because most folks need the cell membrane oil change I told you about.

And when you have had a heart attack or even heart surgery, like stents or bypass, it is even more important to be tanked up on cod liver oil. For like magnesium, it can mean the difference between life and death (Billman, McLennan). You see, **after a heart attack or any heart surgery,** the leading cause of death is not the event or procedure itself. The **leading cause of death is an arrhythmia**. But **magnesium and cod liver oil are among the most crucial nutrients to determine survival, and even negate the arrhythmia from happening in the first place. No drug has the power that these nutrients have** even singularly, much less their combined synergistic survival power.

After coronary bypass surgery atrial fibrillation is a most common complication. Just imagine the poor little heart muscles have been cut into, and deprived of nutrients while on the bypass machine. They should be quivering! Well over 2-dozen studies confirm that **cod liver oil can prevent cardiac arrhythmias and sudden death, after surgery or after heart attacks, and that it does a better job than drugs** (Calo). Instead all sorts of expensive and dangerous cardiology drugs are heroically used in the hospital after these events. But where is the cod liver oil? Where is the magnesium? Where is even a measurement of these? In fact, they should have been measured before the surgery! And this evidential data is over two decades old in dozens of medical journals.

And how does your doctor find out what you need? By simply measuring the fatty acids. But how many cardiologists do this? Not many. In fact if you want to blow his mind, just casually ask if he has measured your EPA (eicosapentaenoic acid) and DHA (docosahexaenoic acid). The look on his face should probably tell you the answer. Yet knowing these values is extremely crucial to not only fixing the cause of your arrhythmia, but also protecting you from future episodes. **It is absolutely imperative to know the levels of fatty acids in the heart, brain, and everywhere** in the body and in even healthy people, much less those who have life-threatening problems.

Evidence:

- Romieu I, et al, **Omega-3 fatty acid prevents heart rate variability** reductions associated with particular matter, *Am J Resp Crit Care Med,* 172:1534-40, 2005
- Schwarz J, et al, **Traffic related pollution and heart rate variability** in the panel of elderly subjects, *Thorax,* 60:455-61, 2005
- Hamade AK, et al, Adverse cardiovascular effects with acute particulate matter and ozone exposures: interest rate variation in mice, *Environ Health Persp,* 116:1033-39, 2008
- Billman GE, et al, **Prevention of ischemia-induced ventricular fibrillation by omega-3 fatty acids,** *Proc Natl Acad Sci, USA,* 91:4427-30, 1994
- Leaf A, **Omega-3 fatty acids and prevention of ventricular fibrillation,** *Prostaglandins Leukot Essent Fatty Acids,* 52:197-8, 1995
- Hallaq H, et al, **Modulation** of dihydropyridine-sensitive **calcium channels** in heart cells **by fish oil fatty acids,** *Prod Natl Acad Sci USA,* 89:1760-4, 1992
- Siddiqui RA, et al, Modulation of enzymatic activities by n-3 polyunsaturated fatty acids to support cardiovascular health, *J Nutr Biochem,* 19:417-37, 2008
- Calo L, et al, **N-3 fatty acids for the prevention of atrial fibrillation** after coronary artery bypass surgery, *J Am Coll Cardiol,* 45:1723-8, 2005
- McLennan PL, et al, Dietary **fish oil prevents ventricular fibrillation** following coronary artery occlusion and reperfusion, *Am Heart J,* 116:709-17, 1988

- McLennan PL, et al, Comparative efficacy of n-3 and n-6 polyunsaturated fatty acids in modulating ventricular fibrillation threshold in marmoset monkeys, *Am J Clin Nutr,* 58:666-69, 1993
- Jahangiri A, et al, Termination of asynchronous contractile activity in rat atrial monocytes by n-3 polyunsaturated fatty acids, *Molec Cel Biochem*, 206; 1-2:33-41, Mar 2000
- Harris WS, Are Omega-three fatty acids the most important nutritional modulators of coronary heart disease risk? *Curr Atheroscler Rep*, 6; 6:447-52, Nov 2004
- Sellmayer A, et al, Effects of dietary fish oil on ventricular premature complexes, *Am J Cardiol,* 76:974-77, 1995

Again the Wrong Suspect is Incriminated

After magnesium, the most commonly ignored cause of arrhythmia is having the wrong fats in the nerve and muscle cell membranes of the heart. Did I say wrong fats? Yes, for we desperately need a fat heart. In fact, the right fats actually talk to our genes and play a critical role in control of every function of the heart. The fats surrounding the nerves are critical for electricity flow as well as for creating the pores or channels in muscles and nerves that regulate the flow of minerals like potassium, magnesium, and calcium that make up the flow of electricity.

Legalized Lying to the Consumer

The tragedy is that your fat status is so easily corrected, yet rarely done. You learned that you want to become experts in avoiding any foods with hydrogenated oils in them (see *Detoxify or Die* for further explanation). For as we referenced in *Total Wellness* newsletter, even **one tablespoonful of trans fats sends over 100,000 damaging molecules to every one of your body's cells**. If the right fats are not in the cell membrane, the electricity cannot flow properly in the nerves and arrhythmia results.

Unfortunately, in order to appease the whining of the food industry as some of the public became knowledgeable enough to avoid trans fats, the FDA it appears to me has legalized lying to you. They did so by passing a regulation in the 2006 *Federal Register* that allowed food manufacturers to plaster **NO TRANS FATS** on the front of a food label if their product contained **500 mg of trans fats per puny half cup serving**. Does this mean the FDA knows (1) what foods you are going to eat, and (2) how much of them, (3) so that your daily total amount of trans fats will not be excessive? Meanwhile, for the unwary, trans fats permeate the food industry disguised in french fries, chips, cookies and crackers, "healthful" salad dressings, breads, condiment sauces, and much more.

And as I have referenced, **Harvard researchers have stated there is no safe level of trans fats**. Now you can also understand why it is so meaningless for states that imposed a "no trans fats" rule in restaurants after this Federal Register decision. It literally has no meaning, plus it has no "teeth". How will they enforce it? Do they know how much of each food you will eat and which foods you will eat each day to be able to ascertain if you have exceeded your "safe" (which has never been determined) level of trans fats?

Trans fats basically put a monkey wrench in your cell membrane chemistry by inserting a fake chemical manufactured by man so that it won't go bad in your pantry. But when this sits in the human cell membrane, it causes serious malfunction, anything from high cholesterol to fatigue and all sorts of arrhythmias in between. Once you get the bad oils out (by becoming very knowledgeable about their hidden sources and avoiding them like the plague that they are), then you need to fix or repair the missing fatty acids to restore the heart to normal electricity, free from arrhythmia.

Rescuing the Starving Heart

When we assay the fatty acids of folks with arrhythmias, or any heart disease for that matter, I find they usually have what I call *the starving heart*. The damaging trans fats are high, but the healing fats, EPA and DHA, are nearly non-existent. **Most folks with arrhythmias need an oil change.** This includes getting the trans fats out of the heart and substituting them with healthful fats that repair the heart's electricity, dependent on its nerves, muscles, mitochondria and blood vessel linings. All of these structures depend heavily on omega-3 fatty acids. You can begin your oil change with one tablespoonful each of **Cod Liver Oil** and **PhosChol,** plus 2 **E Gems Elite,** and one **Gamma Tocopherol** a day for 3-6 months. In addition to magnesium deficiency, fatty acid deficiencies are extremely common and totally correctable leading causes of arrhythmias. Sometimes something as simple as cod liver oil (and don't forget the phosphatidylcholine for the "innards" of the cell membrane sandwich) totally cures an arrhythmia.

Keys to Identifying the "Clueless" Cardiologist

By now you are beginning to appreciate that a cardiologist who fails to immediately focus on your RBC minerals, fatty acids, and vitamin levels is clueless. He has no idea of how to cure you. Move on until you find one deserving of you.

Furthermore, many studies show that arrhythmias after surgeries have been prevented by these nutrients. It's pretty disgusting to me in this era of such sophisticated technology that many in the field of medicine choose to ignore repairing God's basic biochemistry of the human body, yet prefer to dangerously poison the already ailing pathways with drugs. Clearly it's all about money, convenience, speed, ignorance, and not having to understand the chemistry of healing. Let's look at a smattering more of the evidence.

In one study in a high profile cardiology journal of over 11,323 patients who had had a heart attack, those given only one gram of omega-3 fatty acids (as you would find in **a teaspoon of cod liver oil) a day had half the death rate** of those not given it (Marchioli). And **the longer they were on the cod liver oil, the better their survival**. The type used was synthetic and equivalent to less than a teaspoonful of real cod liver oil a day (and of course, this synthetic garbage had none of the vitamins A and D that occur in natural cod liver oil, and I won't bore you with the multitude of other errors in the study). Just think what they could have accomplished by actually measuring all the nutrients and tailoring them to the person's needs! And of course, the researchers didn't even recommend measuring the levels of EPA and DHA so they could figure out the exact amount of cod liver oil needed by each person. Still with such an imperfect study, by **using nutrients instead of drugs they halved the death rate**!

You may find it hard to believe that major **medical journals have shown for over a decade that cod liver oil protects against arrhythmias** (Albert, Sellmayer). Even when researchers looked at all sorts of trials done with inferior doses or synthetic forms, the overall reduction in death was minimum a third less (Bucher). And not only does **cod liver oil reduce arrhythmias** (Leaf, Kang), but **stops restenosis (reclotting) after angioplasty** or roto-rooter (Reis, Kaul, Gapinski, and more in Chapter 5) and **decreases diabetes** (another risk factor for early death) (Feskens), but it also **causes regression or shrinking away of plaque** (Sacks).

So what should we think of a cardiologist or heart surgeon who never mentions the fatty acids like EPA, DHA and trans fats (palmitolaidic), much less assays them? And keep in mind that I'm merely giving you a smattering of the examples and evidence on just a couple of nutrients (out of dozens of them) that have control over arrhythmias (see *The Cholesterol Hoax* for the total protocol). Good or bad, I decided to give you more in depth evidence on a few key nutrients rather than overwhelm you with evidence for every nutrient. And there is lots more overwhelming evidence in the next chapters.

The norm in cardiology seems to be the failure to assay and correct these rudimentary nutrient levels, even in the face of such overwhelming evidence that it should be done. Does this constitute innocent ignorance or blatant stupidity? I let you be the judge, since it's your life that could hang in the balance.

Evidence:

- Studer M, et al, Effect of different antilipemic agents and diets on mortality, *Arch Intern Med*, 165:725-30, 2005
- Bucher HC, et al, N-3 polyunsaturated fatty acids in coronary heart disease: A meta-analysis of randomized controlled trials, *Am J Prev,* 112:298-304, 2002
- Marchioli R, et al, Early **protection against sudden death by n-3** polyunsaturated **fatty acids after myocardial infarction**, *Circulation,* 105:1897-1903, 2002
- Wang C, et al, n-3 Fatty acids from fish or fish-oil supplements, but not a-linolenic secondary-prevention studies: a systematic review, *Am J Clin Nutr,* 84:5-17, 2006
- Leaf A, et al, Membrane effects of the **n-3 fish oil fatty acids, which prevent fatal ventricular arrhythmias,** *J Membr Biol,* 206; 2:129-39, 2005
- Chrysohoou C, et al, Long-term **fish consumption is associated with protection against arrhythmia** in healthy persons in a Mediterranean region – the ATTICA study, *Am J Clin Nutr,* 85: 1385-91, 2007
- Albert CM, et al, Fish consumption and risk of sudden cardiac death, *J Am Med Assoc,* 279:23-28, 1998
- Sellmayer A, et al, Effects of dietary fish oil on ventricular premature complexes, *Am J Cardiol,* 76:974-77, 1995
- Gapinski JP, et al, **Preventing restenosis with fish oils following coronary angioplasty,** a meta-analysis, *Arch Intern Med*, 153:1595-1601, 1993
- Reis GJ, et al, **Randomized trial of fish oil for prevention of restenosis after coronary angioplasty,** *Lancet*, 2:177-81, 1989
- Kaul U, et al, **Fish oil supplements for prevention of restenosis after coronary angioplasty,** *Int J Cardiol,* 35:87-93, 1992
- Sacks FM, et al, Controlled trial **of fish oil for regression of human coronary atherosclerosis,** *J Am Coll Cardiol*, 25:1492-98, 1995
- Feskens EJ, et al, Inverse association between fish intake and risk of glucose intolerance in normoglycemic elderly men and women*, Diabetes Care,* 14:935-41, 1991
- Kang JX, et al, Prevention of fatal cardiac arrhythmias by polyunsaturated fatty acids, *Am J Clin Nutr*, 71(suppl): 202s-207s, 2000
- Falk RH, Atrial fibrillation, *New Engl J Med*, 344; 14:1067-78, 2001

The Clues Don't Add Up:
There's a Tremendous Disconnect in Medicine

Now how about this for a disconnect in medicine. At the Mayo Clinic they reported on a study showing that **cod liver oil is 8**

times more effective in preventing death than defibrillators (Kottke). But still they did not recommend even measuring the levels in a person, much less giving it to cardiology patients. This is in spite of the fact that they stated it cost about $3000 for one defibrillator at a workplace, adding up to $5.2 million dollars to equip U.S. work sites, with an annual replacement cost of $21 million a year. For a defibrillator implanted in your body, the cost is about $101,000 or another $21 million for the projected hypothetical population. This is in contrast to $5.8 million if everyone in a community took cod liver oil daily (or they could eat fish instead of meat with no supplement *ala* Chrysohoou's reference).

So **cod liver oil compared with a defibrillator is 8-times more effective, and well over 4000-times cheaper, not counting all the other health benefits** from healthier cell membranes and other body organs in general. Yet I have not seen any measurement of EPA and DHA fatty acids in any folks on whom I have consulted, who sent voluminous records from the very institutions and clinics where the research was done. Or look at the Harvard study showing **cod liver oil stops arrhythmias** (Leaf). Yet who measures your fatty acids if you go to the cardiology clinic as a patient? Go figure!

And if the cardiologists don't even read their own journals, then for sure the gynecologist isn't going to read them. That is why hormone replacement therapy (HRT) is so often prescribed for post-menopausal women to "protect them from heart disease". This is in spite of the fact that it lowers their level of EPA and DHA, the main fatty acids in cod liver oil (Stark)! That is why HRT was proven to have no protective overall effect for the hearts of women, even though they have been told for decades that it does. In fact it dramatically raises one of their risk factors, CRP, as well as their cancer rate.

Evidence:

- Kottke TE, et al, **Preventing sudden death with n-3** (omega-3) fatty acids and defibrillators, *Am J Prev Med,* 31; 4:316-23, 2006
- Leaf A, et al, Membrane effects of **the n-3 fish oil fatty acids, which prevent fatal ventricular arrhythmias**, *J Membr Biol,* 206; 2:129-39, 2005
- Stark KD, et al, Differential eicosapentaenoic acid elevations and altered cardiovascular disease risk factor responses after supplementation with docosahexaenoic acid in postmenopausal women receiving and not receiving hormone replacement therapy, *Am J Clin Nutr*, 79:765-73, 2004

The Coumadin® Crapshoot

Clearly now you know that anyone treating your arrhythmia should look for all of the curable causes. Unfortunately the norm is to drug, cardiovert and ablate. When cardiologists get nervous that you might throw a clot, they add in the blood thinner Coumadin® (warfarin, a standard rat poison). Or just as ridiculous they tell you to use an aspirin a day. I've dealt with the evidence for these extensively in the books. But the bottom line just for newcomers is that **Coumadin® actually rips calcium out of your bones and dumps it into the coronary arteries**, thereby accelerating arteriosclerosis. It's very counterproductive to your healthful longevity. In the process it triggers bone loss, fractures, osteoporosis, joint replacements and much more.

And **aspirin doubles your stroke and intestinal hemorrhaging risks**, while **the eight parts of vitamin E work much better** and have a litany of beneficial side effects as well for every other part of the body. And when you choose a vitamin E that has all 8 parts, it is even more potent. And lots of other nutrients keep the blood from abnormally clotting, top of which is, you guessed it, **Cod Liver Oil** (Hirai, Tamura), or vitamin B3 in the form of **Niacin Time** (Philipp, Johansson), known for decades.

In one study of just low dose vitamins C, E, beta-carotene, and the mineral selenium, this rudimentary combo not only markedly reduced the ability of platelets to abnormally clump together and clot, but also slashed degeneration and aging of cells (Salonen). No drug even comes close to being able to accomplish this, and that doesn't even count all the other beneficial good "side effects". It's one more good reason (out of dozens) why I often advise folks to add a daily **ACES with Zinc** to their nutrients.

There are many other nutrients as well as food-derived phytochemicals that also turn off unwanted clots. A unique form of aged garlic extract in the form of **Kyolic Liquid** can lower clotting factors like thromboxane B2 and factor IV by 30% (Qureshi, Steiner), while a fermentation product of soybean, called **Nattokinase** also has important fibrinolytic (clot dissolving) properties as well (Sumi, Urano, Fujita). There is so much more to choose from.

Meanwhile, what is your verdict on a cardiologist who prescribes Coumadin®, but never checks your fatty acids, levels of vitamin E (Glynn), intracellular magnesium, fibrinogen, and more? How long will it take for Coumadin® to calcify your coronary arteries and heart valves?

Evidence:
- Price PA, Faus SA, Williamson MK, **Warfarin causes rapid calcification** of the elastic lamellae in rat **arteries and heart valves**, *Arterioscler Thromb Vasc Biol,* 18:1400-07, 1998
- Fiore CE, Tamburino C, Grimaldi D, et al, **Reduced bone mineral content in patients taking an oral anticoagulant**, *South Med J,* 83: 538-42, 1990
- Hirai A, et al, The effects of the oral administration of fish oil concentrate on the release and the metabolism of (14C) arachidonic acid and (14C) eicosapentaenoic acid on human platelets, *Thromb Res,* 28:285-98, 1982
- Tamura Y, et al, Clinical and epidemiologic studies of eicosapentaenoic acid (EPA) in Japan, *Progr Lipid Res,* 25:461-66, 1986
- Glynn R, et al, Effects of random allocation to vitamin E supplementation on the recurrence of venous thromboembolism: report from the Women's Health Study, *Circul,* 116:1497-1503, 2007
- He J, Whelton PK, Vu B, Klag MJ, Aspirin and risk of hemorrhagic stroke; A meta-analysis of randomized controlled trials, *J Amer Med Assoc,* 280; 22:1930-35, 1998

- Philipp CS, et al, Effect of **niacin supplementation on fibrinogen levels** in patients with peripheral vascular disease, *Am J Cardiol,* 82; 5:697-9, 89, September 1, 1998
- Johansen J0, et al, **Nicotinic acid treatment shifts the fibrinolytic balance** favorably and decreases plasma fibrinogen in hypertriglyceridemia, *J Cardiovasc Res,* 4; 3:165-71, June 1997
- Fujita M, et al, **Thrombolytic effect of nattokinase** on a chemically induced thrombosis model in rat, *Biol Pharmacol Bull,* 18; 10:1387-91, October 1995
- Sumi H, et al, A very strong activity of pro-urokinase activator in natural, the traditional fermented soybean in Japan, *Fibrinolysis* 10:31, 1996
- Urano T, et al, The pro-fibrinolytic enzyme subtilisin NAT purified from *Bacillus subtilis* cleaves and inactivates plasminogen activator inhibitor type I, *J Biol Chem,* 276; 27:24690-6, July 6, 2001
- Sumi H, et al, **Enhancement of the fibrinolytic activity in plasma by oral** administration of **nattokinase**, *Acta Haematol,* 84; 3:139-43, 1990
- Steiner M, Li W, *J Nutr,* 131:3s: 980s-4s, 2001
- Qureshi N, et al, *First World Congress on the Health Significance of Garlic and Garlic Constituents,* Washington DC, August 28-30, 1990, page 17 (hundreds of papers available from Kyolic.com)
- Salonen JT, et al, Effects of antioxidant supplementation on platelet function: a randomized pair-matched, placebo-controlled, double-blind trial in men with low antioxidant status, *Am J Clin Nutr,* 53:1222-29, 1991

The Food Factor

And don't overlook simple things like newly emerged food allergies. **A new food allergy can occur in anyone at anytime to anything.** I know thinking of a food allergy is the farthest thing from your mind with life-threatening arrhythmia, but it's a very common cause. Merely eliminating common antigens such as corn (in Scotch) or potato (in vodka) were major in curing several men's end-stage arrhythmias and heart failure. To identify your own food allergies, the cheapest and most thorough way is with the diagnostic diet in *The E.I. Syndrome.*

You Must Render the Verdict

You have enough evidence to be judge and jury. You don't need anyone else when you have an army of men and women from all over the world who have devoted their lives to this research to uncover the mysteries of how God heals the body. Although just a fraction of the evidence, you have all the evidence that you need.

If you have any arrhythmia whatsoever and the cardiologist first wants you to take a drug, or if you are already on drugs and he starts talking about cardioversion or ablation, yet you have had none of these tests, turn around and run out of that room as fast as you can. Medications are great for emergencies and to tide you over until a cure has been found. But be sure there is an educated and dedicated search for that cure.

When you find a cardiologist who wants to measure your RBC magnesium and fatty acids and other nutrients and prescribe the doses that you need, you have hit the jackpot. This guy is going to find and fix what's broken. At least start with the magnesium and membrane repair I've outlined. And this is just a rudimentary beginning. For much more information, how to do all of this in detail, and of course hundreds of references for you and your doctor, start with *The High Blood Pressure Hoax* and then proceed to *The Cholesterol Hoax.*

Solution Sources

For folks who would like one easy source for all of their nutrients in this book, **NEEDS** carries most of these specific brands (www.needs.com or 1-800-634-1380).

Item	Web/Company	800#
Cod Liver Oil, E Gems Elite	carlsonlabs.com	323-4141
Gamma E Gems, ACES w/ Zinc	carlsonlabs.com	323-4141
R-Lipoic Acid, SeaSel, Q-ODT	intensivenutrition.com	333-7414
PhosChol	nutrasal.com	777-1886
Magnesium Chloride Solution (Rx)	windhampharmacy.com	518-734-3033
Natural Calm	supervites.com	888-800-1180
Super Milk Thistle	integrativeinc.com	931-1709
Mag Chlor 85	painstresscenter.com	669-CALM
Cardio/ION	metametrix.com	221-4640
Comprehensive Stool Test	Doctor's Data	323-2784
Kyolic Liquid, Kyo-Chrome	kyolic.com	421-2998
Abx Support	protherainc.com	888-488-2488
Nattokinase	allergyresearchgroup.com	545-9960

Chapter IV

The Mistaken Cases
Of Heart Failure and Cardiomyopathy

Did you know that having a diagnosis of heart failure is worse than having cancer? That is because more people get heart failure in a year than cancer. And worse, they die sooner after the diagnosis. Median survival after the diagnosis of cancer is 6 years. **Median survival after the diagnosis of congestive heart failure is 5 years**. CHF starts with mild shortness of breath, later ankle swelling, then shortness of breath reaches major proportions, limiting walking and even interrupting sleep, then culminates in death.

You'll notice the first two chapters were much briefer. That's because we already have two very complete books on the cure of high blood pressure and cholesterol. The arrhythmia chapter was longer because it's the number one cause of death after someone has had a sudden heart attack, has been in the hospital for a few days, or is a few weeks out past a heart attack (presumably in the recovery phase), or has had heart surgery. Furthermore, arrhythmias can happen without any of those preceding events. I consider the current management of arrhythmias a serious oversight because no drugs cure arrhythmias. Then when cardiologists reached their point of desperation, they resort to electrocuting the heart, often followed by cutting out and throwing away part of it. Cardioversion and laser ablation have become the norm. But where is the norm for looking for the curable causes so you can get rid of the arrhythmia once and for all, and not need to electrocute or ablate?

This chapter will be longer also because (as you just saw) **congestive heart failure (CHF) is worse than having cancer. More people get it each year, and they die sooner once it is diagnosed**. And the same crime occurs. **There are no drugs to cure congestive heart failure**. Yet many folks have been cured of it. An assay of all the biochemistry of the heart allows the physician to find the curable nutrient deficiencies and toxicities, bringing the heart back to normal, as we have done.

CHF folks usually die looking like a walking pharmacy. You learned how hypertension is first treated with diuretics, and then perhaps a beta-blocker (atenolol, as an example), or calcium channel blocker (Norvasc®), or an ace inhibitor (lisinopril). All are common prescriptions loaded with side effects to guarantee worsening. But these few drugs pale in comparison to the categories of drugs used for congestive heart failure. It just supports how desperate the situation becomes when you ignore finding the correctable causes.

The medication categories include any and sometimes all of the following, some of which you have already learned about in the preceding chapters: beta-blockers, calcium channel blockers, digioxin, ACE inhibitors, anticoagulants, nitrates, dopamine, statins, angiotensin II receptor antagonists or blockers, dobutamine, and class III antiarrhythmia drugs. And there's even more. Cardiologists literally pull out all the stops, when it comes to drugs, that is. These all have an arm's length of side effects in the *PDR*, and many more side effects that are not noted, like serious depletion of nutrients that leads to a faster downhill course (Pelton). So let's look at some of the most common causes that are usually overlooked and often curable just by themselves or in combination with other deficiencies and toxicities.

Bill had become a certified couch potato the last year, so short of breath that just walking across the street was tiring. He couldn't remember the last time he dared try a set of stairs. Everything was exhausting, but lifting those legs really showed him he was getting old. Old at 72? He decided to get a diagnosis. His heart was old and failing and he apparently was suffering from a deficiency of drugs, because that is what was prescribed. After a year of mounting pharmacy bills and dwindling heart reserves, he decided to have a peek at his chemistry. Within three months he was off his medications and so healthy that he had both knees repaired and the next year was out dancing.

Congestive heart failure is a mouthful that most have never heard of until they have been slapped with the diagnosis. What it boils down to is a poisoned pump. The heart muscle fibers have become so damaged that they have lost their strength, become swollen and flabby, inflamed, some of them deteriorated or calcified, unable to join together for a unified forceful contraction of blood throughout the blood vessel system.

Over 3 million people suffer from CHF, with over 400,000 new cases diagnosed each year (Bourassa) with half of them dying each year (Ramanathan). In fact, **the chance of living 5 years with CHF is 50%. Even cancer has a better survival rate, and fewer victims**, making CHF a serious silent killer. **Not only is CHF more deadly than cancer, but also its outcome has not improved in 2 decades**. In another study, 6 months after diagnosis 25% are dead, 5 years after diagnosis 67% are dead (Senni, Goldberg). This is a tragic waste of life, in my book a crime.

Evidence:
- Senni M, et al, Mayo Clinic, Congestive heart failure in the community. Trends in incidence and survival in a 10-year period, *Arch Intern Med*, Jan 11, 1999; 159:29-34, Jan 11, 1999
- Goldberg RJ, Univ. Mass., Assessing the population burden from heart failure. Need for sentinel population-based surveillance systems, *Arch Intern Med*, 159:15-17, Jan 11, 1999
- Pelton R, et al, *Drug-Induced Nutrient Depletion Handbook, 2nd Edition*, 1-877-837-5394

A Ubiquitous Culprit:
NSAIDs

Why is there so much CHF? One main reason is it is a common yet silent side effect of very common medications, which nearly everyone has in their home medicine cabinets and gym bags.

NSAIDs are short for non-steroidal anti-inflammatory drugs like Motrin®, Aleve®, ibuprofen, Celebrex®, and even aspirin. There are many more, and as you know, many are over-the-counter, requiring no medical supervision or prescription. In Chapter 1 you learned they are a common yet unsuspected cause of high blood pressure. Worse, NSAIDs cause minimum 20% of hospital admissions for CHF, over 100,000 per year. And they should, because inflammation is a protective phenomenon, just as cholesterol is the Band-Aid for free radical-generated arterial holes. If you axe some of the protective biochemical mechanisms of the body, you pay the price with earlier death.

And the longer you take NSAIDs, the better your chances of destroying heart muscle. **NSAIDs include aspirin that most cardiologists incorrectly recommend to stop unwanted clots.** Please read *The Cholesterol Hoax* so you can educate yourself and your doctor and get off aspirin and on to better alternatives if he has prescribed aspirin for you or himself. If he doesn't read his journals, maybe he reads the newspapers with articles like "Study: Aspirin doesn't prevent first heart attack or stroke" (Oct. 21, 2008, *The Greenville News*, D1).

Meanwhile, there is a 60% increase in the odds of hospitalization for heart failure in folks with no history of heart disease if they have recently used of NSAIDs. **For those who do have a history of heart disease there is a ten-fold increase in risk of hospitalization for heart failure if you use NSAIDs.** And in folks taking long-lasting NSAIDs that last 12 hours or longer there was a 24-fold increase in congestive heart failure risk as opposed to drugs with a half-life of four hours or less. **Aspirin and ibuprofen merely quadruple your risk of heart failure, a four-fold increase** (Page, Heerdink). These authors speculate that prostaglandin inhibition may have something to do with it. But they did not mention leaky gut, loss of nutrients in the work of metabolizing long-term drugs, and a loss of the protective response of inflammation in the heart, much less getting rid of the main causes, heavy metal toxicity and hidden nutrient deficiencies.

By the way if you feel you can't get along without your NSAIDs, think again. Not only do they cause over 100,000 cases of congestive heart failure a year, minimum, and quadruple your heart attack risk, but they also **damage the chemistry of cartilage thereby guaranteeing that you will need a hip or knee replacement** in about 10 to 20 years. If you suffer with chronic pain please read *Pain Free In 6 Weeks* and learn how to find the cause and cure. For many folks, heavy metal toxicity is a big part of the total body burden creating chronic pain.

A large percentage of women take over the family finances. Well, they had better take over the family health, or lose their husbands. Start by getting him off NSAIDs. Lots of nutrients can help, sometimes as simple as a phytochemical from pineapple (bromelain) that has a long track record of dissolving sludge, clots and safely taming inflammation. For starters, **Ananese** is a sublingual form (dissolved under the tongue) that can be titrated to your needs, 2-4 under the tongue, 2-4 times a day.

Evidence:
- Page J, et al, Consumption of **NSAIDs and the development of congestive heart failure** in elderly patients, an under recognized public health problem, *Arch Intern Med*, 160:777-784, Mar 27, 2000
- Heerdink ER, Leufkens HG, Herings RMC, Makker A, et al, **NSAIDs associated with increased risk of congestive heart failure** in elderly patients taking diuretics, *Arch Intern Med,* **1998**; 158:1108-12

Forensics Relies on Many of the Same Clues for Diverse Cases

You learned how important magnesium is for lowering blood pressure, cholesterol and arrhythmias. Well, it is also crucial in heart failure. Since magnesium controls the fluidity of the cell membrane, its deficiency also contributes to the "leaky" blood vessels and fluid retention in ankles of folks with high blood pressure or heart failure (Rayssiguier). Later on the other vessels get leaky and the heart muscle gets weaker, fluid builds up in the lungs, making the victim have to sleep upright in order to avoid shortness of breath (also called orthopnea or dyspnea).

In numerous studies well over half the population is low in magnesium, and these studies looked at the inferior test for magnesium, not the test that shows the truer percentage of deficiency. More modern studies show the average diet gives less than one-tenth of the magnesium folks need (Nielsen evidence in Chapter III). Most cardiology drugs further deplete magnesium, so *the sick get sicker quicker* and require more drugs.

Evidence:
* Rayssiguier Y, Magnesium and lipid metabolism. In Sigel H, Sigel A (eds): *Metal Ions in Biological Systems, Vol 26, Compendium on Magnesium and Its Role in Biology, Nutrition and Physiology*, NY: Marcel Dekker, pp341-58, 1990

A Test to Predict Death Within a Year?

One serious test result for a person with heart failure is an elevated CRP (C-reactive protein). For when this is above normal, it indicates serious inflammation is going on somewhere in the body. What's worse is that **an elevated high sensitivity CRP in a heart failure patient has been shown to be a good predictor that the patient will die within a year** (Berton).

Would you believe that sometimes something as simple and inexpensive as **correcting a hidden magnesium deficiency can lower the CRP**, thereby not only alleviating fatal arrhythmias, but the expected death within 1-5 years from CHF (Almoznino-Sarafian). In fact **low magnesium is commonly found with elevated CRP**. Yet if no one checks either of these, you become a dead statistic. By the way, I don't keep giving you references to magnesium because it is the only mineral to cause these heart problems, for that is not true. I use that example because it is among the most common causes and a perfect example of how negligent drug-oriented or pharmacy-focused medicine is in not checking something so rudimentary, logical and easy, and that has been taught in leading cardiology journals for over two decades.

And dash out the door if your cardiologist prescribes a statin for an elevated CRP. That means he gets his medical information from *The Wall Street Journal* where we learned that CRP is now a Crestor® deficiency (*WSJ*, B1, Nov. 10, 2008) As you can learn in *The Cholesterol Hoax,* an ignored part of vitamin E, gamma tocopherol, is over 300% more effective in lowering CRP, and without the 2 dozen side effects of a statin drug!

Evidence:
- Almonznino-Sarafian D, et al, Magnesium and C-reactive protein in heart failure: an anti-inflammatory effect of magnesium administration?, *Eur J Nutr,* 46:230-37, 2007
- Berton G, et al, C-reactive protein in acute myocardial infarction: association with heart failure, *Am Heart J,* 145: 1094-1101, 2003

The Case of the Poisoned Pump

So what can wear out the cardiac pump? The most common is (1) diet with undiagnosed nutrient deficiencies combined with (2) toxicity, primarily of heavy metals. There are thousands of medical papers documenting the importance of nutrients in correcting heart failure, from CoQ10 (poisoned by statin cholesterol-lowering drugs), carnitine (poisoned by the plasticizers in our bodies), phosphatidyl choline (lowered by membrane damage from a trans fatty acids diet), D-Ribose, and other nutrients as well as nearly every vitamin, mineral, fatty acid, amino acid and more.

When it comes to environmental pollutants, everything from diesel exhaust to plasticizers, Teflon, trans fats, fire retardants, lead, mercury (from fish, dental fillings, exhausts from power plants and more), arsenic (in chicken, pressure treated lumber, cigarettes, and more), aluminum (from baked goods, processed foods, coffee makers, drinking water, and much more).

For the naysayers, let me just quickly remind you that we all have this stuff in us, even newborn babies and animals in the pristine wild. Government reports show that we have so poisoned the world that even the polar bears in the arctic have hypothyroidism and osteoporosis from our chemicals. Environmental toxins, the invisible enemy, are a major cause of our epidemics of diseases occurring at progressively younger ages (see *Detoxify or Die* and *Total Wellness* for evidence and disease-reversing treatment*)*.

Is Your Doctor Handcuffed?

There is a very disturbing disconnect in medicine that I cannot understand. What I mean by this is that even if you go to the prestigious clinics where some of the most important groundbreaking research has been done, if you go to their cardiology clinic for treatment, it is as though they are totally ignorant of the research that was done right under their roof, in their own institution. Don't they talk to each other? Don't they read their own medical journals? It's as though they are wearing blinders.

One example from the famed Mayo clinic showed they studied end-stage heart failure patients, for whom nothing else could be done. Medicine had nothing more to offer. They were exceedingly short of breath and maximally medicated. Life was limited. Researchers put them in a special sauna. I say special because when someone has CHF, even a heat wave or a hot bath can kill them, so a regular sauna would be out of the question.

But in the special sauna, they got rid of enough of these modern chemicals, which silently damage the heart, that they reversed their heart failure. **They did with a special detox sauna what nothing else in medicine could do**. They normalized the CHF patients' blood pressure, lowered their shortness of breath, improved the strength of the heart pump (improved ejection fraction measured by the cardiologist), they dropped several drugs, were happier and healthier. They accomplished by reversing their congestive heart failure what no drug could. Yet with all the consultations I have done on folks whose records included an evaluation at the Mayo Clinic, nowhere was the **far infrared sauna** suggested or discussed, much less recommended. And this was done over a decade ago. Now how do you figure that happens?

For a complete description of how to do this special sauna, where to get it, and of course, the evidence from top cardiology journals, read *Detoxify or Die*. And your detoxification does not end there, because heavy metals like mercury, cadmium, lead and more also contribute to poisoning the calcium channels, heart nerves and heart muscles. You need to also get rid of mercury and other heavy metals (Bemis), all described in *The High Blood Pressure Hoax*).

Evidence:
- Tei C, Horikiri Y, Park JC, Tanaka N, et al (Mayo Clinic), Acute hemodynamic **improvement by thermal vasodilation in congestive heart failure**, *Circulation,* 19:2382-90, 1995
- Bemis JC, et al, Polychlorinated biphenyls and **methylmercury alter intracellular calcium** concentrations in rat cerebellar granule cells, *Neuro-Toxicol*, 21; 6:1123-34, 2000

Forensics:
Did the Victim Need a Thiamin Boost?

How do we get low in vitamin B1 (thiamin)? Poor diet, alcohol, and a host of medications like diuretics prescribed for heart failure or hypertension (Seligmann). Another sneaky cause is a gut full of the yeast Candida, from previous antibiotics or a sweet tooth. This yeast in the gut can make an enzyme to destroy thiamin called **thiaminase, thus creating a silent B1 deficiency that builds and leads to fluid retention and heart failure.**

Meanwhile, refractory heart failure, resistant to all that medicine can offer has been turned around with pennies of this B1 vitamin, but only if the treating cardiologist thinks of it (Shimon, Mendoza). **But Vitamin B1, thiamin, is deficient in over a third of patients with CHF** (Hanninen). And this is just looking at the blood level, not the organic acids which show a functional level: translation, there is a better test that even shows if, in spite of taking it, your particular genetic make-up requires you to take more than average to keep your heart healthy. Clues for your doc that you need more than the average person are elevated pyruvate, disproportionate lactate/pyruvate, a-ketoisovalerate, a-keto-isocaproate, and a-keto-b-methylvalerate on the **Cardio/ION Panel**.

I have never seen a cardiac case (and I've seen them from most of the major cardiology clinics in the U.S.) whose records showed anyone ever thought of it. The dose I would suggest is 1 a day of **Vitamin B1** 100 mg, as well as many of the other items you will learn about. **The chance that it is due to just one thing is very slim**. But curing heart failure depends on finding all the missing elements that result in the full orchestration of health. Meanwhile, vitamin B1 is extremely inexpensive, frequently deficient, and harmless as a trial. Even a glass of wine a day can increase your need, not to mention the plethora of environmental pollutants we continually fend off each day.

And at the risk of repeating myself, I must remind you that everything you learn about heart disease also helps you be a better detective for finding the causes and cures for other forms of heart disease. **Sometimes thiamine cannot normalize until a magnesium deficiency is corrected** (Zieve), or the diuretic is replaced by curing the blood pressure. For many others a thiamine deficiency is sustained because they have an overgrowth of yeast in the intestines called *Candida albicans* **that secretes the enzyme thiaminase that destroys vitamin B1** before it even gets a chance to get absorbed. This yeast overgrowth is often triggered by a diet high in sweets, alcohol, sodas, or in folks who have had antibiotics or steroids. You need to diagnose and cure that (for more information on the causes and cures of Candida read *No More Heartburn*).

Evidence:

- Zieve L, Influence of **magnesium deficiency on the normalization of thiamin**, *Ann NY Acad Sci*, 162; 732-43, 1969
- Rogers SA, Using organic acids to diagnose and manage recalcitrant patients, *Integrative Medicine*, 5; 4:52-61, Aug/Sep 2006
- Hanninen SA, et al, The prevalence of thiamin deficiency in hospitalized patients with congestive heart failure, *J Am Coll Cardiol*, 47:354-61, 2006
- Seligmann HG, et al, Thiamin deficiency in patients with congestive heart failure receiving long-term furosemide therapy: a pilot study, *Am J Med*, 91; 2:151-5, 1991
- Shimon I, et al, **Improved left ventricular function after thiamine supplementation in patients with congestive heart failure** receiving long-term furosemide therapy, *Am J Med,* 98:485-90, 1995
- Mendoza CE, **Reversal of refractory congestive heart failure after thiamine** supplementation: report of a case and review of the literature, *J Cardiocasc Pharmacol Therapeut,* 8; 4:313-16, 2003

One of the Desperation Moves

When things get really desperate, expensive injections of Natrecor® (nesiritide) are given in hopes of prolonging the survival of the heart failure victim. This hormone, the result of genetic engineering, is made to resemble our own natriuretic hormone. So how could we make more of our own? With one of the forgotten parts of real vitamin E, gamma tocopherol.

One major problem is cheap vitamins that only list "vitamin E" are really not vitamin E, which contains 8 isomers or parts. If it says "vitamin E', then it is probably only alpha tocopherol, and often synthetic to make matters even worse. For when you take only the alpha part of vitamin E, it actually lowers your gamma tocopherol level, and when your vitamin E is synthetic, it even lowers the level of any good or real vitamin E from your foods (Ohrvall, Jiang).

Meanwhile, (one of the eight parts of real vitamin E,) **gamma to-copherol is a natriuretic hormone, meaning it makes the kidneys excrete sodium** (Uto-Kondo, Yoshikawa, Jiang). You want to bet the Natrecor® injection is expensive and it only lasts maximum 3 hours. The smart cardiologist would have checked your gamma tocopherol level when you were first seen and made sure it and alpha tocopherol were in the top quintile (more on that in *The Cholesterol Hoax*), thus sparing you much of this life-robbing and expensive misery. You can start with adding 1 **Gamma E Gems** to your daily program of 1-2 **E Gems Elite**.

Isn't it amazing that every place you look, God has provided what we need through food and nutrients? Meanwhile, it now will not surprise you that if you look at the levels of gamma tocopherol in folks who have any type of heart disease, including recent heart attacks, their levels are about four times lower than folks without heart disease (Ohrvall, Devaraj, Dietrich, Jiang). In fact, it now turns out that your **gamma tocopherol level is a better marker of coronary heart disease than something as useless as the cholesterol level** (Jiang, McCarty). And remember from *Total Wellness* and *The Cholesterol Hoax*, it does lots more like tame cancer cells and lower CRP. Luckily gamma tocopherol is only part of the crystal ball test that shows you your other cardiovascular risk factors, plus what needs repairing so that you can heal the heart. More on that later.

Meanwhile, do not forget that everything you learn about finding the clues for curing and healing is applicable in new situations. For example, **magnesium is also important in regulating the sodium pump** that is in the cell membrane of every heart cell. The magnesium level is just as important in congestive heart failure as it is for high blood pressure, high cholesterol, or arrhythmia cures.

Evidence:

- Uto-Kondo H, et al, g-Tocopherol accelerated sodium excretion in a dose-dependent manner in rats with a high sodium intake, *J Clin Biochem Nutr,* 41:211-17, Nov 2007
- Cachs JR, et al, Interaction of magnesium with the sodium pump of the human red cell, *J Physiol,* 400:575-91, 1988
- Yoshikawa S, et al, The effect of g-tocopherol administration on a-tocopherol levels, and metabolism in humans, *Europ J Clin Nutr,* 59:900-05, 2005
- Ohrvall M, et al, Gamma, but not alpha, tocopherol levels in serum are reduced in coronary heart disease patients, *J Intern Med*, 239:111-17, 1996
- Devaraj S, et al, Failure of E in clinical trials: Is gamma-tocopherol the answer?, *Nutr Rev,* 63;8:290-93, 2005
- Dietrich M, et al, Does g-tocopherol play a role in the primary prevention of heart disease and cancer? A review, *J Am Coll Nutr,* 25; 4:292-99, 2006
- Jiang Q, et al, g-Tocopherol and its major metabolite, in contrast to a-tocopherol, inhibit cyclooxygenase activity in macrophages and epithelial cells, *Proc Nat'l Acad Sci*, 97; 21:11494-99, Oct 10, 2000
- Jiang Q, et al, g-Tocopherol, but not a-tocopherol, decreases proinflammatory eicosanoids and inflammation damage in rats, *FASEB J,* 17:816-22, 2003
- McCarty MF, Gamma-tocopherol may promote effective NO synthase function by protecting tetrahydrobioptin from peroxynitrate, *Med Hypoth*, 69:1367-70, 2007

Fat's Where It's At

And speaking of cell membranes, by now you know that any cardiologist pretending to treat you without assaying and fixing your cell membrane chemistry hasn't a clue of how to get you well. A healthy cell membrane is imperative for it contains, among other crucial regulators, all the mineral/ion pumps i.e., for sodium (instead of that wretched salt-free diet), calcium, potassium (instead of those awful stomach-irritating capsules and powders), magnesium, and more. In fact supplementing the right fatty acids cuts the death rate and hospitalizations for heart failure by over 8%. **Cod liver oil is far superior to statin drugs that are routinely prescribed** (O'Riordan, GISSI-HF, Fonarow).

Clearly the evidence is now overwhelming. **No one should prescribe statins in heart failure**, because they don't help. Furthermore, cod liver oil does help reduce death between 2-20% (GISSI-HF). And that doesn't count the inevitable worsening on statins from all the side effects. But **cod liver oil was over 10 times more helpful.** And these docs didn't even measure it or balance it with all the other missing nutrients! Plus nutrients when harmonized have the potential to cure!

Evidence:
- O'Riordan M, **Omega-3 fatty acids, but not statin therapy, cuts mortality and hospitalizations in heart failure** (http://www.medscape.com/view article/579983)
- Fonarow GC, **Statins and n-3 fatty acid supplementation in heart failure**, *Lancet,* 372 (9645): 1195-96, Oct. 2008
- GISSI-HF investigators, Effect of n-3 polyunsaturated fatty acids in patients with chronic heart failure (the GISSI-HF trial): a randomized, double-blind placebo-controlled trial, *Lancet*, 372: 1223-30, Oct. 4, 2008

The Heavy Metal Clue

Rare is the person with congestive heart failure who does not have hidden heavy metal poisoning. To safely detoxify your lead and other heavy metals from your body that not only create heart failure, but hypertension, coronary plaque, arrhythmias and more, you may have heard you need chelation. But be aware that there is a method that is 5 times safer, and cheaper than chelation, and it is done with non-prescription items. For full details, proceed to *The High Blood Pressure Hoax.* Since we're all loaded with heavy metals, it's only a matter of time before we get some form of degenerative disease attributed to "old age". That's why even if you don't have any heart disease yet, you want to start on a detoxification program. For starters these heavy metals have a large bearing on who gets cancers, and especially cancers that eventually become resistant to all forms of chemotherapy and radiation. As well, heavy metals rot and deteriorate the brain, but we erroneously chalk that also up to old age.

Definitely you want to get your **Cardio/ION** first to determine your deficiencies and correct them. **You never want to try to detoxify before you have repaired some of the outstanding deficiencies that got you sick in the first place**. Besides that, chelating out heavy metals takes months and years, but once you are on the path, the improvement is usually steady. You just continue to get stronger. To go to an even higher level of wellness after that, proceed to *The Cholesterol Hoax*. Also *Total Wellness* newsletter keeps you abreast of current findings above and beyond the books and in between future books.

Evidence:

- Navas-Acien A, et al, Lead exposure and cardiovascular disease-A systematic review, *Environ Health Persp*, 115; 3:472-82, 2007
- Shih RA, et al, Cumulative lead dose and cognitive function in adults: a review of studies that measured both blood lead and bone lead, *Environ Health Persp,* 115; 3: 43-92 March 2007

Quick Fixes to Keep the Victim Off the Morgue Slab

In the meantime, what can you do *today* to improve your heart failure? Luckily there are many nutrients that are lacking in the failed heart. So the odds are with you that you will stumble onto a combination that can lift your energy, breathing ability and spirits immediately. Let's take a look at some of these nutrients, what they do, and the evidence for them. Bear in mind that **it is assumed that you are already taking the nutrients that you have learned about in the preceding chapters here.** Heart failure is so serious that it is a rare person who doesn't also have severe magnesium deficiencies along with multiple mineral, fatty acid, vitamin, and other nutrient deficiencies.

I have chosen to look at a few nutrients that you may not be as familiar with, as they are even more rarely prescribed, but crucial for restoring vitality to a failing heart. I'm going to give you an example of just three of what I call "orphan" nutrients, as examples of many nutrients that have been proven crucial in reversing conges-

82

tive heart failure. What boggles the mind is that with all of this data (and I'm only presenting a smattering of it), where are the cardiologists who are using these nutrients? Better yet, they could be doing the proper blood tests to determine more precisely not only what you need, but also how much you need. Let's look at these three examples. Then you decide.

The CoQ Question

I thought every man on the street knew about CoQ10, yet I rarely hear of a cardiologist who is measuring it, or even prescribing it. Since it's so harmless and helps shuttle the electrons through the mitochondria so that energy can be created in the failing heart muscle, why isn't it used? Even whole books have been written about CoQ10, much less hundreds of medical papers. The scary part is that at **least two major categories of cardiology drugs create a CoQ10 deficiency.** This is even all the more reason why every cardiologist should be measuring it and supplementing it.

Both **statin drugs for cholesterol and the beta-blockers for angina, arrhythmias, hypertension, and more, lower CoQ10. They actually** poison part of its synthetic pathway in the body (Folkers, Kishi). For example with the statin drugs, by poisoning the enzyme that makes cholesterol in the liver, HMG- CoA reductase, unfortunately that enzyme also makes CoQ10. That's why many people on statin drugs go on to develop congestive heart failure, tooth loss, fatigue, depression and other symptoms of CoQ10 deficiency. And it has been known for well over a decade that if you give CoQ10 when you have someone on a statin drug, you can prevent loss of CoQ10 and resultant heart problems (Berger). In fact the evidence is clear: **it is highly recommended to give CoQ10 to anyone on a statin drug to decrease the chance of introducing CoQ10 deficiency symptoms.**

But how many doctors who prescribe statin drugs also prescribe CoQ10? Clearly any cardiologist who knows anything about the

83

mechanism of the drugs that he is licensed to prescribe should at least be measuring the CoQ10 levels if someone has any heart problems, or especially if he has put them on either of these two categories of drugs. **He may have actually worsened their congestive heart failure**. Certainly he has the power to reverse it.

Meanwhile, CoQ10 is like a train that shuttles electrons back and forth inside the mitochondria. In every heart muscle and nerve cell are little bean-shaped organelles called mitochondria. This is where energy is made. If there is insufficient CoQ10, then you can make energy until the cows come home, but there is no delivery system for it.

Because there are often so many nutrients to take in order to repair the damaged heart, whenever we can bypass a capsule or pill form I like to do it. That's why my favorite form of CoQ10 is an <u>o</u>ral <u>d</u>issolving <u>t</u>ablet that is absorbed under the tongue. Use 2-3 **Q-ODT** sublingually (under the tongue with no food or drink for 20 minutes before or after) twice daily for starters.

Evidence:

- Folkers, K, Longsjoen P, Willis RA, et al, **Lovastatin decreases coenzyme 10 levels in humans**, *Proc Natl Acad Sci*, 87:8931-34, 1990
- Kishi T, et al, Bioenergetics in clinical medicine XV. Inhibition of coenzyme Q10-enzymes by clinically used alpha adrenergic blockers of beta-receptors, *Rev Commun Chem Pathol Pharmacol*, 17:157-94, 1977
- Sinatra ST, **Refractory congestive heart failure successfully managed with high-dose coenzyme Q10** administration, *Molec Aspects Med*, 18: S299-305, 1997
- Berman M., et al, Coenzyme Q10 in patients with end-stage heart failure awaiting cardiac transplantation: a randomized, placebo-controlled study, *Clin Cardiol*, 27:294-99, 2004
- Khatta M, et al, The effect of coenzyme Q10 in patients with congestive heart failure, *Ann Intern Med*, 132:636-40, 2000
- Hoffman-Bang C, et al, **Coenzyme Q10 as an adjunctive in the treatment of congestive heart failure,** *Am J Cardiol*, supple 19; 3:2168, 1992
- Baggio E, et al, Italian multi-center study on the safety and efficacy of coenzyme Q10 as adjunct therapy in heart failure, *Molec Aspects Med*, 15 (supple): 287-94, 1994

- Berger AM, et al, Exogenous CoQ10 supplementation prevents plasma ubiquinone reduction induced by HMG-CoA reductase inhibitors, *Molec Aspects Med,* 15 (supple): 187-193, 1994
- Morisco C, et al, Effect of coenzyme Q therapy in patients with congestive heart failure: a long-term multi-center randomized study, *Clin Investig,* 71 (supple): S134-136, 1993

Should You Boost Your Heart's Fuel Pump?

Would you own a beautiful car without a fuel pump?   Why would anyone want to be caught in the predicament of having plenty of fuel, but unable to get it to the engine? Yet that is what the body is like without sufficient carnitine. For it moves the main fuel for the heart muscle into the mitochondria. This is where God's miracle occurs turning fat from foods into energy that runs every cell. Carnitine literally piggybacks the fats into the mitochondria, the small kidney bean-shaped area inside of cells where energy is made. **Without carnitine, the fats (fuel) cannot get inside cellular mitochondria to be converted to energy**. And heart muscle without energy is called congestive heart failure.

It is downright scary how little mainstream medicine knows about the scientific literature of the last two decades that can save lives, more importantly after everything that drug-driven medicine and pharmacy-focused physicians can offer has failed. I just don't understand the reticence to use safe, proven natural remedies, especially when they have no side effects and no known adverse interactions with any medications. Just check back at the dates of these research articles to prove to yourself how negligent and ignorant "modern" cardiology appears to me.

Carnitine meets the criteria to be called a vitamin, because it is synthesized by the body from an amino acid (just as the vitamin niacin (B3) is synthesized from tryptophan). But still underappreciated and not even officially recognized as essential, it is what I term an orphan nutrient.

Carnitine has reversed angina and reduces the ST-depression (the EKG sign of serious angina that will lead to heart attack). As well, **it has reversed congestive heart failure as well as reduced the number of drugs** needed. Carnitine has **speeded recovery after heart attack**, made the victim require less anti-arrhythmia drugs and other heart medication, **lowered cholesterol and triglycerides**, and **reduced arrhythmias**. It has even improved intermittent claudication (which you can think of as angina of the legs, where instead of chest pain and shortness of breath with walking, you get leg pains that inhibit walking).

And as is true of any good nutrient, you do not have to be sick to benefit from it. **Carnitine has improved the exercise tolerance of seasoned athletes and weakened weekend warriors**. Yet it is powerful enough to improve the exercise tolerance of chronic lung patients. And it has helped conditions as diverse as Alzheimer's and senile depression to Down's syndrome and dialysis patients. Diabetics have greatly benefited from the improved health of blood vessels as well as nerves, two areas badly damaged by the disease.

There is no medication that can do all that, and without side effects. But that is not all that carnitine can do. It is crucial to a recovering liver, and stops chemotherapy drugs, like adriamycin commonly used in breast cancer, and AZT used for HIV, as examples, from one of their most lethal symptoms, killing the heart. And don't forget that **many stents are coated with a form of chemotherapy in the attempt to reduce clotting**. But where are the cardiologists who measure and supplement carnitine to reduce both events? And **carnitine helps the alcoholic liver heal**. It has even corrected low sperm counts and decreased sperm motility on fertility testing. And on the other end of the spectrum it has even helped athletes improve stamina, since they can move fatty acids into the mitochondria quicker to create more energy.

But why does a person get low in carnitine and how can they tell if they are low? Carnitine deficiency is extremely common because

86

the number one pollutant in the human body, plasticizers poisons the ability of the body to make sufficient carnitine. Clearly we cannot get away from plasticizers (phthalates), because they outgas into our foods, from plastic water bottles, infant formula and soda bottles, food packaging, home furnishings, construction materials, medications (especially time release or slow release or extended release formulations), computers, wiring in homes, appliances, and much more. So use **Acetyl L-Carnitine Powder**, 500-1000 mg twice a day for starters.

Phthalates, the pollutant from plasticizers (**over 10,000 times higher than any other pollutant in our bodies**) is so high in our bodies that it damages a lot more than just carnitine. That's why it's essential to get it out, especially if you have any resistant disease. The directions are in *Detoxify or Die*. For many resistant heart diseases from high blood pressure too high cholesterol, angina, arrhythmias or even coronary artery calcifications, **just getting the phthalates out has been curative**. And congestive heart failure is no exception.

Evidence:

- Ghidini O, et al, Evaluation of the therapeutic efficiency efficacy of **L-carnitine** in **congestive heart failure**, *Internat J Clin Pharm Therapeut Toxicol,* 26; 4:217-20, 1988
- Martin MA, et al, Myocardial **carnitine** and carnitine palmitoyltransferase deficiencies in patients with **severe heart failure**, *Biochim Biophys Acta,* 1502; 3:330-36, 2000
- Sethi R, et al, Beneficial effects of propionyl-L-carnitine on sarcolemmal changes in **congestive heart failure** due to myocardial infarction, *Cardiovasc Res,* 42; 3:607-15, 1999
- Suzuki Y, et al, Myocardial **carnitine deficiency in chronic heart failure**, *Lancet,* 1; 8263:116, 1982 (**over 27 years ago in a leading heart journal**)
- Cerchi A, et al, Effects of L-carnitine on exercise tolerance in chronic stable angina: A multicenter, double-blind randomized, placebo controlled crossover study, *Int J Clin Pharm Ther Tox,* 23:569-72, 1985
- Bartels GL, et al, Effects of L-propionylcarnitine on ischemia-induced myocardial dysfunction in men with angina pectoris, *Am J Cardiol,* 74:125-30, 1994

- Davini P, et al, Controlled study on L-carnitine therapeutic efficacy in post-infarction, *Drugs Exp Clin Res,* 18:355-365, 1992
- Dragan AM, et al, Studies concerning some acute biological changes after exogenous administration of 1 g L-carnitine in elite athletes, *Physiologie,* 24:231-234, 1987
- Pettegrew JW, et al, Clinical and neurochemical effects of acetyl-L-carnitine in Alzheimer's disease, *Neurobiol Aging,* 16:1-4, 1995
- Furitano G, et al, Polygraphic evaluation of effects of **carnitine in patients on Adriamycin treatments**, *Drugs Exp Clin Res,* 10:107-111, **1984**

Is Your Cardiologist Guilty of Your Slow Death by CHF?

He is if you haven't had a trial of the nutrients in this entire book, and of course a measurement of these nutrients to determine precisely what you need. Bare minimum you need the **Cardio/ION Panel** to assess the biochemical/nutritional status of the damaged, failing heart. And I have seen many remarkable recoveries from CHF (off medications, no longer short of breath, out dancing, golfing without a cart, strong enough to have knee replacements, etc.), but most of them also needed an intensive heavy metal detox program, as described in *The High Blood Pressure Hoax.*

As an example of the importance of this test, I'll repeat: The plasticizers from our plastic water and soda bottles and that permeate our air, food and water in a multitude of ways are the number one pollutant in the human body. Plasticizers are over 10,000 times higher than any other pollutant. **We are the first generation of man to ever have such an unprecedented level of chemicals in our bodies.** One of the many damages that the **plasticizers do is destroy the carnitine synthesis.** In fact **knowing the carnitine levels is actually a marker for congestive heart failure** (El-Aroussy). Yet if a doctor does not assay your organic acids to see an **elevated adipate, suberate or ethylmalonate, or EPA/DHA, how will he know that you have a carnitine deficiency?** So he will miss a golden opportunity to cure your congestive heart failure or at least find one more of the missing ingredients needed to bring you to that cure. He is working blindly. Do you really want a blind cardiologist?

And all these nutrients are integrally related in a delicate balance. For example, carnitine can influence taurine levels (the number one amino acid in the heart, and is also a magnesium facilitator, stabilizes the cell membranes, **reduces homocysteine**, promotes diuresis, stops clots and more, (see *The High Blood Pressure Hoax*). Taurine, in turn has reversed CHF in folks. It all depends on your individual deficiencies and needs, which every doctor is privy to via the **Cardio/ION**.

Evidence:
- El-Aroussy W, et al, **Plasma carnitine levels as a marker of impaired left ventricular functions**, *Molec Cell Biochem*, 213 (1-2): 37-41, 2000
- Azuma J, et al, Taurine for treatment of congestive heart failure, *Int J Cardiol*, 2; 2:303-4, 1982
- Sanderson SL, et al, Effects of dietary fat and L-carnitine on plasma and whole blood taurine concentrations and cardiac function in healthy dogs fed protein-restricted diets, *Am J Vet Res,* 62; 10:1616-23, 2001

D-Ribose Rescues Hibernating Heart Tissue

What makes the world go round? Is it love? Is it money? Whichever it is, these are the currencies, if you will, the driving forces. The driving force in the human body is a molecule of energy called ATP (adenosine triphosphate). It's one of God's many miracles where he has designed our chemistry so that it converts molecules of food into ATP. This energy currency, ATP, in turn runs everything in the body. One of the problems with congestive heart failure is the heart muscle can't make enough ATP to keep it running. Just how much does it take?

The heart uses more energy per its weight than any other organ in the body. The heart contains about 700 mg of ATP, which is only enough to drive 10 heartbeats. Since we average about 90,000 heartbeats a day, we consume over 6000 g of ATP. This is all made inside the mitochondria and you already learned **how important it is to fix the mitochondrial cell membranes with the oil change.** So if we take a peek at a molecule of ATP (which I know you have been eager to do), we will see that sitting smack dab in the center of it is a sugar called ribose.

One of the many problems of the failing heart is that it just cannot make as much energy as fast as it is needed. That's why victims have to pace themselves and cannot overdo. D-Ribose however, a naturally occurring sugar in the human body, has been shown in many studies to **rev up the production of energy**. It does it in the sickest of folks with congestive heart failure and on the other end of the spectrum in elite athletes. It is crucial for recovering quicker after a heart attack, and improves angina and high blood pressure. Plus carnitine **even makes nonfunctioning heart muscle cells (called hibernating) start producing energy and contracting normally again. It rescues "dead" heart muscle!**

For the seasoned athletes, D-Ribose speeds up recovery time during and after stressful competitions and it lessens downtime after workouts that have produced soreness. On the flip side of the spectrum, for those who are in the throws of a heart attack, **ribose helps preserve the function of the rest of the heart cells during the heart attack** (Befera).

I suggest, the best form being **Corvalen,** a heaping scoop twice a day for starters. And for any naysayers who don't know anything about the chemistry of it and think that it might be toxic or have some negative attribute, just remind them: in the many studies that have been done, they all show there is **no adverse effect** (Griffiths). After all it is a normal metabolite in the human body. So start using it to find out whether you have some heart muscle "playing possum". It may appear dead merely because it needs D-Ribose to rescue and resurrect hibernating muscle cells.

Evidence:

- Omran H, et al, **D-ribose aids congestive heart patients**, *Exp Clin Cardiol,* 9; 2:117-18, 2004
- Vijay N, et al, Ventilatory efficiency **improves with D-ribose in congestive heart failure** patients, *J Molec Cell Cardiol,* 38; 5:820, 2005
- Carter Old, et al, **D-ribose improves peak exercise capacity and ventilatory efficiency in heart failure patients**, *J Am Coll Cardiol,* 43 (3 suppl A): 185a, 2005
- Griffiths JC, et al, Sub-chronic (13-Week) oral toxicity study with D-ribose in Wistar rats *Food Chemical Toxicology,* 45:144-152, 2007,
- Omran H, et al, D-Ribose improves diastolic function and quality of life in congestive heart failure patients: A prospective feasibility study, *Europ J Heart Fail,* 5; 5:615-19, Oct. 2003
- Illien S, et al, **Ribose improves myocardial function in congestive heart failure**, *FASEB J,* 15; 5:A142, 2001
- Sharma R, et al, D-ribose improves doppler TEI myocardial performance index and maximal exercise capacity in stage C heart failure, *J Molec Cell Cardiol,* 38; 5:853, 2005
- Gradus-Pizlo I, et al, Effect of D-ribose on the **detection of the hibernating myocardium** during the low dose dobutamine stress echocardiography, *Circul,* 100; 18:3394, 1999 (**rescues "dead" hearts, 10 years ago!**)
- Befera N, et al, Ribose treatment helps preserve function of the remote myocardium after myocardial infarction, *J Surg Res,* 137; 2:156, 2007
- Ingwall JS, et al, Is the failing heart energy starved? On using chemical energy to support cardiac function, *Circul Res,* 95; 2:135-45, 2004
- Omran H, et al, **Ribose improves myocardial function and quality of life in congestive heart failure patients**, *J Molec Cell Cardiol,* 33; 6:80-173, 2001

The Universal Alibi

To forget D is **D**umb. Do you recall how vitamin D (cholecalciferol) is crucial for hypertension, hyperlipidemia, keeping calcium off coronaries, and halving your heart attack rate? Well it is also important in congestive heart failure (Zittermann). Even Harvard clinicians/researchers have shown many references on how a low vitamin D contributes to heart failure (Giovannucci). Instead drugs loaded with side effects are used to bludgeon the symptoms that vitamin D can prevent or reverse (like CHF, abnormal renin-angiotensin, coronary calcifications, hypertension and heart attacks). And remember in various studies **40-100% of folks have unsuspected vitamin D deficiencies. It is literally epidemic.** Furthermore studies have shown that 10,000 IU for six months has been very safe (Vieth). Take at least 1-2 **Solar D Gems** 2000 mg daily (Aloia). Meanwhile, always remember all your knowledge about each case is cumulative in helping you solve others that may seem unrelated. **Nutrients are the tools with which the body heals**. It was designed that way.

Remember **the universal alibi in medicine is that malpractice is defined as not doing what the herd (local standard of care) does**. Right or wrong, regardless of evidence and deaths, you are free from hassles if you do what the next guy does. If the practice guidelines (many of whose designers benefit financially from the pharmaceutical industry) say every disease is a deficiency of a drug, then so be it. Then just open any prestigious medical journal, like *The New England Journal of Medicine*. You have to plough through multiple ads before you get to a medical article. What does the first half contain? Drug ads. And what funds much of the university research presented? Pharmaceutical companies. And what are most of the articles about? How the latest drug stops some symptom. Hogwash to actually curing things with cheap nutrients that a patient can buy without a doctor's help. It pales in comparison to looking like a hero with an expensive prescription-only, exotic-sounding, "magical" drug.

Evidence:
- Zittermann A, et al, Low vitamin D status: a contributing factor in the pathogenesis of congestive heart failure*? J Am Coll Cardiol,* 41:105-12, 2003
- Zittermann A, Vitamin D and disease prevention with special reference to cardiovascular disease, *Progr Biophys Molec Biol*, 92:39-48, 2006
- Vieth R, Why the requirement for vitamin D3 is probably much higher than what is officially recommended for adults. *J Steroid Biochem Molec Biol*, 89-90:575-9, 2004
- Aloia JF, et al, Vitamin D intake to attain the desired serum 25-hydroxyvitamin D concentration, *Am J Clin Nutr*, 87:1952-58, 2008
- Giovannucci E, et al, 25-Hydroxy-vitamin D and risk of myocardial infarction in men, *Arch Intern Med*, 168; 11: 1174-80, 2008

The Cardiomyopathy Conundrum

When cardiologists are really stumped about what's causing your congestive heart failure they often make a diagnosis of cardiomyopathy, which merely means a severely poisoned heart. CHF folks need an even more intense detox protocol, beginning with *Detoxify or Die* for the plasticizers and other environmental chemicals, then progressing to *The High Blood Pressure Hoax* for the heavy metal aspect, and culminating in *The Cholesterol Hoax* for fine-tuning. I would suggest reading the monthly newsletter, *Total Wellness*, as well since we continually put new findings in there, again complete with all the scientific evidence. I haven't figured out a way to do it any cheaper and as completely for folks who need immediate life-saving repair.

Meanwhile, every nutrient we talked about here for congestive heart failure is equally important in cardiomyopathy folks. For example, many times something as simple as carnitine has started to turn them around. Of course, they have many deficiencies and usually one or more severe toxicities for sure. The good news is even a heart that is poisoned has rallied, even though the majority of cardiologists tell folks "There is no known cause and no known cure".

For those ready for a quantum leap, I'd like to give you just a glimpse of one tiny example of the many powerful tools I've explained in more detail in *TW* and the books. **Copper is crucial to recovery of the heart with cardiomyopathy** (Madeiros). In fact when researchers want to create cardiomyopathy for experiments, they can merely create a copper deficiency (Kopp)   Sadly, a lot of this data goes back over three decades. So there's really no excuse for any cardiologists being ignorant of it. Yet when was the last time you heard of someone on death's doorstep with cardiomyopathy having an RBC copper measured? I never have in 39 years of medical practice.

Three quarters or **75% of the heart muscle cell is totally made up of the mitochondria.** And think about it. It has to be since it's the main energy machine of the body. For cytochrome-C oxidase plus superoxide dismutase and lysyl oxidase are three important copper containing enzymes that have to be plentifully supplied with copper in order to keep this energy machine, your heart, beating for its over 87,000 times a day, every day for all the years of your life.

In fact when the enzyme lysyl oxidase becomes deficient in copper, the blood vessels and heart muscles lose their elasticity and become arteriosclerotic (Seyama). In a nutshell, when copper becomes secretly deficient, conditions like congestive heart failure or cardiomyopathy or arrhythmias are diagnosed, but are bludgeoned to death with pharmaceuticals. Meanwhile those "healthful" packaged fruit juices loaded with high fructose corn syrup and pasteurized (kills all the vitamins), then "fortified" with synthetic nutrients, are one of the many triggering factors for a copper deficiency (Reiser).

Since copper can really upset your stomach, and it lowers zinc (which is already lowered by plastics in your environment, most medications, and the American diet) I searched for the most well tolerated copper/zinc, combination that also gave good blood levels. I recommend at least one a day of **Zinc Balance** (Jarrow).

Meanwhile, an interesting device that we have recommended (and referenced) for years works by actually revving up this important enzyme, **cytochrome-C oxidase**. But a copper deficiency can be a main reason to keep it from doing its "magic" (references in *TW* 2005-7). This device is so potent that in experiments giving mice methanol or wood alcohol that invariably causes blindness, those with the **Lumen** over their eyes did not become blind. We've used it successfully and repeatedly on many folks for rescuing teeth from extraction or root canal, for reducing the recovery time from knee, back, hip, and shoulder injuries from weeks to days, and more. I wonder what it would do for the heart?

Evidence:

- Paulson DJ, **Carnitine deficiency-induced cardiomyopathy**, *Molec Cell Biochem,* 180; 1-2:33-41, 1998
- Rizos I, Three-year survival of patients with heart failure caused by dilated cardiomyopathy and L-carnitine administration, *Am Heart J,* 139; 2 Pt 3:s120-123, 2000
- Asai T, et al, Combined therapy with PPARa agonist and L-carnitine rescues lipotoxic cardiomyopathy due to systemic carnitine deficiency, *Cardiovasc Res,* 70; 3:566-77, 2006
- Madeiros DM, et al, Newer findings on a unified perspective of copper restriction and cardiomyopathy, *Proc Soc Exp Biol Med,* 250:299-313, 1997
- Kopp SJ, et al, Physiologic and metabolic characterization of the **cardiomyopathy induced by chronic copper deficiency.** *Am J Physiol,* 245: H855-66, 1983
- Madeiros DM, et al, A unified perspective on **copper deficiency and cardiomyopathy**, *Proc Soc Exp Biol Med,* 203:262-73, 1993 (**Over 16 years ago!**)
- Reiser S, et al, **Dietary fructose exacerbates the cardiac abnormalities of copper deficiency in rats**, *Atherosclerosis,* 74:203-14, 1980 (**Over 29 years old!**)
- Segame Y, et al, Atherosclerois and matrix dystrophy, *J Atheroscler Thromb,* 11: 236-45, 2004

Chemotherapy-Induced Cardiomyopathy

One of the most common causes of cardiomyopathy are drugs, while chemotherapeutic agents for cancers, rheumatoid arthritis, colitis, severe asthma and other autoimmune diseases lead the pack. The sad thing is for years in *TW* we have published some of the many studies to prove that giving various antioxidant nutrients, the very ones you have learned about in this book, actually keep chemotherapy drugs from killing the heart or causing cardiomyopathy. And these nutrients not only save the heart from chemotherapy-induced death (a leading cause of cancer death), but also even make the chemotherapy work better. Instead unknowledgeable oncologists tell folks not to take any nutrients because it will interfere with the action of chemotherapy. This is not true and we've given the evidence many times over the years from successful oncologists all over the world. In fact, it is one of the primary foci of *TW* in future issues, as well.

The Myocarditis Mystery

Medicine loves to mystify you and put you off the trail by throwing a medical term your way that has little actual meaning. Myocarditis is one such term, for it is merely a cover-up for the fact that cardiologists haven't a clue about what is causing your heart tissues to be wildly inflamed and slowly dying. Sadly myocarditis (and cardiomyopathy as well as pericarditis or pericardial effusion translated as fluid around the heart) progressively happens more often in young folks, well under 50. When medicine is stumped, the universal alibi is conveniently pulled out of the hat, "It's caused by a virus". Most of these folks have the same pathology: serious heavy metal toxicities and nutrient deficiencies, just like the others here. The difference is merely that it's usually proceeding at a faster pace. Consequently, it is more emergent that the victims become quickly involved and highly informed. Many die because they procrastinate to see what the "experts" would do first. It's easier.

Is IV Chelation Necessary?

Now if your condition is emergent, you could use IV chelation to get rid of the heavy metals that we all silently spend a lifetime stocking up on. But it has drawbacks; (1) mainly that it is expensive (over $150 a session), (2) time-consuming (often 2-4 hours 2-3 times a week), and folks (3) frequently need to travel miles to find a practitioner.

Worst of all, (4) it further loads the body with its number one body toxin, phthalates. They outgas from the IV tubing and bag, adding to the metabolic damage to an already ailing body (Barry, Roth,

Loff, *DOD*).   **Plasticizers from IVs can also be a major reason folks go downhill after long hospitalizations.** In addition, (5) after each chelation session most physicians administer a "canned" dose of "corrective" minerals, a one-dose/size-fits-all type of thing, sort of like pantyhose. When we see the actual blood levels of these folks they are miserably low, which explains their symptoms. (6) The high dose most often used has killed kidneys and patients.

Infinitely safer, less expensive, easier and non-prescription is the heavy metal detox protocol spelled out in detail, which uses a rectal suppository at night of the same chemical as the IV, and an even stronger oral capsule of a different form of heavy metal detox for day time (**NOT SIMULTANEOUSLY**), and more. This protocol is much safer, **over 5 times cheaper, non-prescription, done at home, and with doses tailored to your individual system's tolerance**.

If you need proof of your toxicities, you can have your cardiologist prescribe the **Porphyrin Test** (described further in *The Cholesterol Hoax*) and do the **Heavy Metal Provocation Test** (described in *The High Blood Pressure Hoax*) that prove that heavy metals as well as plasticizers and other pollutants are part of the hidden causes of your heart failure. For this is curable, yes, reversible; concepts that cardiology does not normally associate with congestive heart failure. But for my money I'd rather have you spend your dollars on getting the **Cardio/ION,** since I've never seen a case of CHF that didn't have toxicities. Why spend money proving the toxicities that we all have? Better to determine the nutrients you need so that you can more safely and efficiently detoxify.

One huge advantage of the Cardio/ION is that it enables your cardiologist to look at the whole "elephant" at once. Some doctors look at one aspect like fatty acids, then months later the minerals, and months later the vitamins, etc. The bigger the whole picture at once, the greater the opportunity to diagnose what you're dealing with. It's analogous to being shown a 2" photo of various parts of an elephant, versus the whole elephant at once to decide what kind of animal it is. In my opinion, the twelve pages of the Cardio/ION give the best overall view to enable you to most clearly identify "the elephant".

Evidence:
- Barry YA, et al, Perioperative exposure to plasticizers in patients undergoing cardiopulmonary bypass, *J Thorac Cardiovasc Surg*, 97:900-05, 1989
- RothB, et al, Di-(2-ethylhexyl)-phthalates as a plasticizer in PVC respiratory tubing systems: indications of hazardous effect on pulmonary function in mechanically ventilated preterm infants, *Europ J Pediat Surg*, 147:41-6, 1988
- Loff S, et al, Polyvinyl chloride **infusion lines exposed infants to large amount of toxic plasticizers**, *J Pediat Surg,* 35:1775-81, 2000

What Can You Do Today?

Forget about solving the crime for now. Sure you could ask your cardiologist what he knows about CoQ10, D-ribose, gamma tocopherol, carnitine, thiamin, copper, or cholecaliciferol. But why aggravate yourself!? There is enough time for interrogating him in the next chapters. Instead protect yourself so that you are not the next victim. If you have congestive heart failure, you need to get going and start saving your own life first. You need to start today!

*If you are totally new to the idea of curing your own heart failure, at least start with the easy 1-2-3 of magnesium and membrane repair in the previous chapters and then add in **Acetyl-L-Carnitine, Solar D Gems, Corvalen, Q-ODT,** and **Vitamin B1.** When you have caught up enough on your reading, start the far infrared sauna protocol in* Detoxify or Die *to begin to get the underlying environmental toxins out of your heart that reverse even end-stage congestive heart failure, just as the Mayo Clinic studies did. You can render your verdict later on this **unsolved crime**. Right now you have to concentrate on reading and living. It would be a tragic shame for you to die now. Just when you are starting to learn that your disease is reversible!*

Solution Sources:

For folks who would like one easy source for all of their nutrients in this book, **NEEDS** carries many (needs.com or 1-800-634-1380).

Item	Web/Company	800#
Vitamin B1 (100 mg), E Gems Elite	carlsonlabs.com	323-4141
Gamma E Gems, Solar D Gems	carlsonlabs.com	323-4141
Acetyl L-Carnitine Powder	carlsonlabs.com	323-4141
Cardio/ION, Porphyrin	metametrix.com	221-4640
Heavy-metal provocation	metametrix.com	221-4640
Corvalen (D-Ribose)	integrativeinc.com	931-1709
Q-ODT, Ananese	intensivenutrition.com	333-7414
Far infrared sauna	hightechhealth.com	794-5355
Far infrared sauna	saunaray.com	877-992-1100
Zinc Balance	jarrow.com	634-1380
Lumen	lumenphoton.com	828-863-4834

Chapter V

After Your First Heart Attack and/or Stent, You Must Terminate Progression, Angina, Plaque, and Coronary Calcifications

The Magnesium Clue Continues to Provide Evidence

What must you do when you have a heart attack? You want to insist on magnesium. In one study, they gave every other victim who entered the emergency room with a heart attack 750 mg IV of magnesium (Rasmussen). Those who got this small dose of magnesium (very inadequate if they were low enough to have a heart attack to begin with) had half the arrhythmias that folks who didn't get magnesium had. Nearly 50% of the people who did not get magnesium had an arrhythmia. And you must recall that **arrhythmia is a major cause of death after a heart attack**. But only 21% of folks who got the magnesium daily had arrhythmias (and they were grossly under-dosed plus no other nutrients were checked or given). Still, I'd rather have one in five odds versus one in two for a life-threatening arrhythmia.

Furthermore, **for those who got this inadequately small token dose of magnesium, only 7% died, whereas nearly triple the amount 19% died who did not get magnesium**. The sad thing is the study was done 20 years ago and the emergency room docs still don't give it routinely in the emergency room or direct it to be given in the ambulance. And this is among hundreds of papers proving that magnesium increases your chances of survival dramatically. In fact **magnesium status is a major determinant of who walks out of the hospital in a few days versus who is carried out in a body bag**. And don't forget the studies that show that **nearly everyone who enters the hospital for whatever reason is deficient in magnesium**. And other studies prove many other minerals and other nutrients are deficient as well. There just is no money to be made in giving people nutrients. Pharmaceutical profits drive medicine (see the 3 books for political evidence that is beyond what I want to burden you with here).

Here is an example of some of the questions answered in our monthly newsletter, *Total Wellness*, further documenting how pervasive the ignorance of magnesium deficiency is.

Q. *When I had a heart attack, on the way to the hospital I asked for a shot of magnesium in the ambulance and in the emergency room, since you showed how it increases survival. I was refused in both places. When I got my Cardio/ION, which was done prior to my heart attack (but results were not back yet), I had been deficient in magnesium all along. When I checked my hospital records, after discharge, no magnesium was ever checked. How do we protect ourselves against such ignorance?*

A. That is exactly why I continue this newsletter in its 20th year and continue to put out the books with the latest data and instructions. Right now **the average daily intake of magnesium in the USA**, land of plenty and with the world's most expensive medical system (but not the best health care), **is 70-100 mg a day.** And (depending on which institutions' stats you read) **the pathetic RDA is only around 300-400 mg**. If that were not bad enough, add this scary fact: **As the RBC magnesium goes down, the body tries to compensate, so the serum magnesium** (the inferior, insensitive one that should never be used) **goes up** (Nielsen). So the guy who orders the inferior one will feel even more confident that he is doing good medicine and that you are O.K.

Meanwhile, recall **normal serum magnesium is so worthless that you can walk out of the office and have a heart attack any moment due to magnesium deficiency.** If that were not enough, **low magnesium is a key cause of arrhythmias, angina, high blood pressure, congestive heart failure, insulin resistance, diabetes, high cholesterol, osteoporosis, depression, insomnia, migraines, asthma, irritable bowel, and more. Get bare mini-**

mum, 600 mg a day if not 1000 or more (review Chapter 1 and more in *The Cholesterol Hoax*). Many folks titrate to their symptoms. They know immediately if they are low in magnesium because they get muscle cramps, eye twitches, angina or other symptoms they use as a barometer. As you can see, you had better stay tanked up on magnesium, (1) to prevent another heart attack, and (2) to be on the protected side if you do have one. Right now, however, you need to identify and rectify the causes of your attack.

Evidence:

- Nielsen FH, et al, Dietary magnesium deficiency induces heart rhythm changes, impairs glucose tolerance, and decreases serum cholesterol in post menopausal women, *J Am Coll Nutr*, 26; 2:121-32, 2007
- Rasmussen HS, Clinical intervention studies on magnesium in myocardial infarction, *Magnesium,* 8:316-25, 1989
- Canon LA, et al, Magnesium levels in cardiac arrest victims: **relationship between magnesium levels and successful resuscitation,** *Ann Emerg Med,* 16, 1195-98, 1987
- Whang R, Ryder KW, Frequency of hypomagnesemia and hypermagnesemia, requested versus routine, *J Amer Med Assoc,* 2634; 3063-4, 1990

Just the Tip of the Iceberg

You now are an expert in one of the primary minerals in the heart, magnesium. The point is not to even suggest that magnesium is the most important or the only important nutrient. The point is to make you an expert in an example of one of a staggering array of nutrients needed for healing the "impossible". They are enormously powerful when orchestrated together, and tailored to your needs. For example, by understanding how important magnesium is (as just one example of one mineral) in healing every condition of the heart, **it becomes mind-boggling to understand why your cardiologist has failed to order an intracellular magnesium**. Yet even though it has been the sole cause of many folks' cardiac conditions, it is more likely that you have multiple deficiencies, not just a solo one.

Clearly, **the more nutrients you become proficient in, the greater your armamentarium of healing tools**. As you accumulate knowledge in more nutrients and then ultimately in detoxification as well, you'll see that you can heal just about anything. It doesn't have to be restricted to the heart. And this healing is even when everything that medicine has to offer has failed, or you've been told there is *"no known cause"* or *"no known cure"*. The more you learn, the more you are able to see right through those ridiculous pronouncements. When you hear *"You've had every test there is"* or *"We've done everything possible"*, you are now able to decide if that is true or not, or whether there is more to the story.

Angina's Warning Clue

Regarding magnesium, when folks have angina, it's often due to spasm of a coronary artery. It actually squeezes down so there is less blood flow and consequently less oxygen to the heart muscle. This causes lactic acid build-up and the pain or heaviness, just as any muscle is painful when there's not enough blood supply. You can just tie a tourniquet around a finger to see how painful lack of oxygen can be. Many nutrients you have already learned about, like **Vitamin B1, R-Lipoic Acid or D-Ribose, can speed up the clean-up of lactate.** And, **oftentimes just correcting the magnesium will terminate angina.** Let's look at some of the evidence.

In one study, just giving **magnesium cut coronary artery pain after exercise by as much as 21%** (Shechter). But you must be sure that you are in the top quintile (the top or high side of "normal") on the assay. For many people with angina caused by magnesium deficiency need as much as 1000 mg or even 2000 mg or more of magnesium a day. This could put them way above the "normal" level. But so-be-it. That is what their bodies require to function optimally now. However once the rest of their nutrients are assayed and balanced, then their kidneys don't waste so much magnesium and they require a lot less. Also remember, if all else fails, most people need to get the lead, mercury, cadmium, or other heavy metals out of their kidneys in order to stop wasting or losing magnesium (directions for all of this are in *The High Blood Pressure Hoax).*

Bear in mind that all these aids you are learning about are crucial for every aspect of heart disease. For example, after surgery for aortic valve repair, D-Ribose, **Corvalen**, can keep you from going into heart failure and being bludgeoned with drugs (Vance).

Evidence:
- Vance R, et al, D- ribose maintains ejection fraction following aortic valve surgery, *FASEB J*, 14; 4: A419, 2000
- Shechter M, et al, Effects of oral magnesium therapy on exercise tolerance, exercise-induced chest pain, and quality of life in patients with coronary artery disease, *Am J Cardiol,* 91:517-21, 2003

The Case of the Misplaced Calcium

Some folks put their calcium in all the wrong places: they make kidney stones, gallstones, they calcify tendons or make calcific spurs in their backbones, knees, hips, heels or shoulders. Others dump their calcium in the toxic waste site of the body. They plaster it onto the brain or coronary arteries (Meema, Leonard). Whenever you have misplaced calcium, you know you had better check the magnesium first and actually do the whole **Cardio/ION** panel, for your chemistry is severely dysfunctional.

There is also an inexpensive test that you can get without a prescription that shows calcifications in your coronary arteries, but without the danger of dying from someone injecting a radioactive dye into your arteries, as in an arteriogram or angiography. This test is done with x-ray technique within less than a few minutes. In fact you don't even have to take your clothes off. You may be lucky enough to have someone in your area who does the Coronary Calcium Score via an ultrafast heartscan.

If you don't have anyone in your area that does the ultrafast heartscan, the best deal is in Florida. Nearly everyone has an excuse to go there, either for a business meeting, a professional conference, to visit a relative there, or take the kids to Disney World. You can schedule yourself without a prescription by merely calling **Diagnostic Outpatient Centers** 1-800-890-4452 and schedule your **coronary calcium score by ultrafast heartscan** either in Orlando (Leesburg, Ocala, and Eustis) or the alternative office in St. Petersburg (between Tampa and Sarasota). Be sure to ask for the discount that is given to Dr. Sherry Rogers' readers.

For around a couple hundred dollars you have the same information that your friends are getting from angiography where they are hospitalized and given anesthesia (from which they could die), injected with a foreign material that the body never completely gets rid of and has caused autoimmune diseases. Plus they paid well over $1000 for this chance of dying. But you don't even take your clothes off and it takes less than 10 minutes and is 5 times less expensive and non-prescription.

You will **know how much calcium is in your coronary arteries**, and in fact in which arteries and how much. And as we've seen time and again, your cholesterol level has hardly any bearing at all. Folks who never had high cholesterol have elevated coronary calcium scores, while folks with sky-high cholesterol for years have totally clean arteries. That's one more reason why the test is so important. **The coronary calcium score indicates how much time you have before a heart attack**. And best of all you have the opportunity to markedly slow down and even *reverse* the calcifications (see *The Cholesterol Hoax*). The same test is available for the arteries on the way to your brain (carotids), and much more. You cannot afford to miss having this "crystal ball" test.

After the Heart Attack or Stent:
Melt Your Plaque and Get Rid of the Cause

In *The Cholesterol Hoax,* I showed you there the uncontroversial evidence **that aspirin-recommending cardiologists are archaic** in their lack of knowledge if they are prescribing aspirin or taking it themselves. Well, if they won't believe all of the evidence from the top cardiology journals, perhaps they will believe a recent study by Harvard Medical School researchers done on over 39,000 patients.

They showed that taking **vitamin E supplements produced a 21% lower risk of blood clots,** including deep vein thrombosis of the legs and pulmonary emboli of the lungs. High-risk folks like **women who had already had blood clots, had an even better reduction in risk, 44%** (Glynn). The 600 mg of natural source vitamin E a day did produce a slightly higher risk of nosebleeds, but it was a lower risk than low-dose aspirin produced (and the study's E was unbalanced with all 8 parts of vitamin E).

If they can't **believe Harvard that natural vitamin E is better than aspirin made from a petrochemical,** what would it take for them to get on board the 21st century medicine train? Another study showed that **400 IU of vitamin E cut the risk of cardiovascular disease by more than 50%** in diabetics. You recall diabetics have four times the risk of early heart disease as compared with the average person, and that some folks need as much vitamin E as 3200 IU/day, depending on their chemistry, and that this is proven to be a very safe level (Roberts). Obviously the greater the number of complementary, harmonizing antioxidants you have on board, like vitamin C to make E even more effective, the lower can be your level of vitamin E (much more in *The Cholesterol Hoax* and *TW*).

Evidence:

- Glynn RJ, et al, Effects of random allocation to vitamin E supplementation on the occurrence of venous thromboembolism. Report from the Women's Health Study, *Circulation,* 116:1497-1503, 2007
- Roberts LJ, et al, The relationship between dose of vitamin E and suppression of oxidative stress in humans, *Free Rad Biol Med*, 2007

Oil Those Arteries So Plaque Slips Right Off

I've told you a lot of the benefits of cod liver oil in the preceding chapters. Clearly after folks have had a heart attack, cod liver oil prevents restenosis (re-clotting of the artery), plus it reduces the chance of heart failure and arrhythmias. Because it keeps folks from clotting off their new stents, and much more, I have to warn you about misleading studies. I'll just give you one example.

In this one (which I hope your cardiologist doesn't use as evidence for keeping you off cod liver oil), they found that fish oil did not help reduce death or heart attacks or arrhythmias or congestive heart failure following a heart attack. You would think that this would be an important study. But it's not. In fact it's totally flawed. The patients were on a slew of drugs. You can't hope to override the effect of drugs sucking nutrients out of an already damaged body by just giving back one nutrient. Let's look at the drugs among these average patients; 85% of patients were on aspirin, 60% were on beta-blockers, 10% were on ACE inhibitors, and 68% were on statins. What chance did they have of healing with all those medications dragging nutrients out of their bodies faster than they could put them back in (Nilsen)? Furthermore, and lots of these studies are run by folks who just don't do enough studying, they used inferior quality and/or synthetic nutrients. Truly the devil is in the details, and so is the cure.

Clearly, if you have had a heart attack, a stent, other cardiac surgery, or have calcifications of the coronary arteries, you should be on **Cod Liver Oil.** There is no excuse for not taking it, as it comes in capsules, lemon-flavored liquid, children's doses, and even as tasteless, aroma-less **Fish Oil**. It is so neutral in this form that we put it on popcorn at a meeting, and no one knew. For my money, I would be on the best form I could find, ethically made by dedicated people. Furthermore, in this era of such sophistication where we send people to the moon, it's inconceivable to me that any cardiologists would fail to measure your actual fatty acids to determine the precise balance needed by your individual body. Just look at a smattering of the decades of evidence.

Evidence:
- Nilsen DW, et al, Effects of high-dose concentrate of n-3 fatty acids or corn oil introduced early after acute myocardial infarction on serum triacylglycerol and HDL cholesterol. *Am J Clin Nutr,* 74:50-56, 2001
- Gapinski JP, et al, **Preventing restenosis with fish oils following coronary angioplasty**, A meta-analysis, *Arch Intern Med,* 153:1595-1601, 1993
- Reis GJ, et al, **Randomised trial of fish oil for prevention of restenosis after coronary angioplasty,** *Lancet,* 2:177-81, 1989
- Kaul U, et al, **Fish oil supplements for prevention of restenosis after coronary angioplasty,** *Int J Cardiol,* 35:87-93, 1992
- Sacks FM, et al, Controlled trial **of fish oil for regression of human coronary atherosclerosis,** *J Am Coll Cardiol,* 25:1492-98, 1995
- Albert CM, et al, Fish consumption and risk of sudden cardiac death, *J Am Med Assoc,* 279:23-28, 1998
- Sellmayer A, et al, Effects of dietary fish oil on ventricular premature complexes, *Am J Cardiol,* 76:974-77, 1995

There is Something Fishy About This Evidence

You have learned how important repairing the heart cell membranes is to preventing heart problems as well as healing them after the fact. The basic recipe is (1) eliminate the trans fat from the diet, (2) measure the fatty acids so you know precisely how much correction is needed, (3), repair the cell and mitochondrial membranes with the proper amounts of **Cod Liver Oil, PhosChol**, and all eight parts of vitamin E; the best way for doing this is with 1-2 **E Gems Elite** plus one **Gamma E Gems** daily as well as 1-2 **Tocotrienols** twice a day.

Follow this recipe if you cannot afford to do the blood test, since this corrects some of the most commonly assayed deficiencies. You will probably find it is unbelievable, as I did that in this era, that most cardiologists do not yet measure the most important part of the heart, the cell membrane where all the receptors are and all the communication messages originate from. Yet they have no qualms about poisoning these very receptors every day with calcium channel blockers, beta-blockers, ACE inhibitors, angiotensin blockers, and many more membrane poisons. Incredible!

In one review article from Tufts New England Medical Center in Boston, they reviewed well over 100 papers in the literature and found that consuming fish or **fish-oil supplements markedly reduced sudden cardiac arrest**. In fact, cod liver oil reduced the risk of death just from all types of heart disease as well as other non-cardiac diseases in some studies **by as much as 50%.** There's no drug that does that. And for sure drugs are not as safe or inexpensive, plus drugs don't fix anything.

And the ignorance of the researchers in many of the food studies was astounding because they never even differentiated whether fish was fried with trans fatty acids or not, which of course dilutes the overall results. Other researchers looked at fish consumption in folks in as much as 36 countries at once, obviously overlooking the fact that the results of the US would certainly be less advantageous, because we eat more junk food and more processed foods with trans fatty acids and additives that counter the good effect of fish than many other cultures (Wang). Meanwhile, **numerous studies prove fish oil and other nutrients have much more power than drugs.** For example, **fish oil reduced heart death risk by 32% whereas statins only 22%** (Struder).

Furthermore, many studies showed that **you could prevent or dramatically slow down restenosis with cod liver oil after coronary angiography, a heart attack, angioplasty or stents.** An added benefit is that cod liver oil does not increase bleeding like the dangerous conventional anticoagulants do. For remember, medicines like **Coumadin® pull calcium out of the bones making you more prone to fractures and osteoporosis. Worse, they dump the calcium into the coronary arteries, making you more prone to further heart attacks**. That's why I feel if you had any of these procedures done and your cardiologist does not measure your levels of EPA and DHA, trans fats and other fatty acids and recommend cod liver oil, I would recommend you cross examine him to find out exactly why not. And what exactly does he plan on doing to reduce your recurrence? I think you might be surprised by his answers now that you know so much.

Evidence:
- Wang C, et al, n-3 fatty acids from fish or fish-oil supplements, but not a-linolenic acid, benefit cardiovascular disease outcomes in primary-and secondary-prevention studies: a systematic review, *Am J Clin Nutr,* 84:5-17, 2006
- Struder, Briel, et al, Effect of different antilipidemic agents and diet on mortality, *Arch Intern Me*d, 165:725-30, Apr 11, 2005
- Kaul U, et al, **Fish oil supplements for prevention of restenosis after coronary angiography,** *Internat J Cardiol,* 35:87-93, 1992
- Maresta A, et al, **Prevention of post-coronary angioplasty restenosis by Omega-3** fatty acids: main results of the Espent for Prevention of Restenosis Italian Study (ESPRIT), *Am Heart J, 143*: E5, 2002
- Dehmer GJ, et al, **Reduction in the rate of early restenosis after coronary angioplasty by a diet supplemented with n-3 fatty acids**, *New Engl J Med*, 319:733-40, 1988
- Franzen D, et al, Prospective randomized double-blind trial on the effect of **fish oil on the incidence of restenosis following PTCA**, *Catheter Cardiovasc Diagn,* 28:301-10, 1993
- Eritsland J, et al, Long-term effects of n-3 polyunsaturated fatty acids on hemostatic variables and bleeding episodes in patients with coronary artery disease, *Blood Coag Fibrinol,* 6:17-22, 1995
- Leaf A, et al, Do **fish oils prevent restenosis** after coronary angiography?, *Circulation,* 90:2248-57, 1994
- Miller MR, et al, Usefulness of **fish oil supplements in preventing clinical evidence of restenosis after percutaneous transluminal coronary angiography**, *Am J Cardiol*, 64:294-9, 1989

- Cairns JA, et al, Fish oils and low molecular weight heparin for the reduction of restenosis after percutaneous transluminal coronary angiography, *Circulation,* 94:1553-60, 1996

Can You Catch a Heart Attack?

What an absurd idea. Or is it? Lots of common bugs get in the body and can live there for years with no symptoms. Meanwhile they silently burrow into the coronary arteries. The body sends a cholesterol patch to stop any leakage, but cardiologists bludgeon the cholesterol with a statin, rather than looking for the underlying cause and curing it.

Sometimes it is as simple as the antibiotic doxycycline to get rid of *Chlamydia pneumoniae* that has lingered there since a flu or bronchitis years ago. For folks who doubt such could happen, realize that **79% of carotid artery plaque has antibodies to Chlamydia, while only 4% of arteries without plaque have antibodies** to this common bug (Muhlstrin).

Even though it may be a new bug to you, this bug isn't that rare, as many folks have already encountered it as a flu with coughing, sneezing and sometimes a bronchitis or pneumonia. But now scientists find that *Chlamydia can burrow into the walls of blood vessels lingering there for years,* creating a steady inflammatory reaction. It becomes a nidus or focal point for infection; a "sore spot" that attracts repair cells that use cholesterol as a patch. When the patch becomes large enough, it becomes a clot that blocks the flow of blood to the rest of that vessel. If it is in a heart vessel, this becomes a heart attack. If the clot breaks off and floats to another vessel, such as the brain, a stroke results. Meanwhile these pear-shaped microbes can get a free ride inside white blood cells (macrophages) indefinitely (details, diagnosis and treatment in *The Cholesterol Hoax*).

.

H. pylori is even worse, because it's an even more common bug, and more deadly. This bug even creates cancers. **Two out of every three people have this bug silently living in their stomachs.** For some it causes no symptoms, or in others a little heartburn. For others it rots out the lining of the stomach so that they don't make enough hydrochloric acid. The result of this atrophic gastritis is that they don't absorb their nutrients. Consequently, they age rapidly and die of multiple undiagnosed nutrient deficiencies.

And the acid-inhibiting drugs used for heartburn and H. pylori can create B12, zinc, and magnesium deficiencies, for starters (Ruscin, Ozutemiz, Epstein). Yet, when folks no longer absorb B12, they get symptoms that mimic Alzheimer's. For lack of a blood test and pennies of B12, many have been warehoused for life with Alzheimer's. And you have already learned a smattering of what devastation low magnesium and zinc cause. And the drugs inhibit the absorption of a lot more, but you get the idea. In addition, this bug, which grows even faster when you take acid-inhibiting non-prescriptions (like prilosec) or prescription drugs (like Nexium® that you learned about earlier), also can cause stomach cancer. In fact it's one of the few cancers that can be cured with an antibiotic, because when they killed the bug, the cancer went away.

Meanwhile this bug silently burrows its way into the bloodstream and for some reason makes a beeline for the coronary arteries. When it sets up housekeeping there, it actually drills holes in the walls of the coronary arteries. But again our bodies are designed to protect themselves, so cholesterol comes along to patch up the holes. However, in keeping with its *modus operandi*, modern medicine bludgeons this cholesterol with a statin drug, loaded with side effects that include other diseases and cancers. This merely amounts to **shooting the messenger**. It does nothing to cure the underlying cause. Meanwhile, sometimes a simple phytonutrient like **Kyolic Liquid** can actually kill the bug, while other times triple antibiotics are needed (see *No More Heartburn* for more details).

This isn't the first time that infectious agents have been linked to heart disease. Viruses like herpes simplex, cytomegalovirus and coxsackie-B virus have caused cardiomyopathies and myocarditis. These are just big words for serious enlargement and/or inflammation of the heart that can lead to heart failure and death. And we have known for decades that streptococcal infections in the teeth or elsewhere can get into the bloodstream and attack heart valves, resulting in damage that requires surgical repair or synthetic valve replacements. But the key is why is this particular heart vulnerable to bugs that nearly everyone has been exposed to? The answer is now obvious. These folks are not playing with a full deck of nutrients plus they carry too heavy a chemical burden.

Luckily there are many nutrients (like vitamins D, C, E, EFAs, etc.) as well as phytonutrients (like lutein, zeaxanthin, lycopene, silymarin, aged garlic, etc,) plus factors derived from organisms (like beta glucan, lactoferrin, colostrums, etc.) that improve the bug-fighting ability of the body. As one small example **NSC-24 Beta Glucan Circulatory Formula** revs up the macrophages (white blood cells) in their ability to fight infection and sometimes prevents infections by 30%. That's only one reason why some folks choose to use it prophylactically, since it can also lower the accumulation of plaque on arterial walls, mitigate unwanted clotting, and more.

Or look at **Kyolic Liquid** with hundreds of studies worldwide, a proprietary aged garlic, that not only fights Candida and H. pylori, but attenuates progression of coronary plaque (Budoff), clots, blood pressure, cholesterol and much more, with only a couple of squirts a day. Or use your detox cocktail and **SeaSel,** (selenium) and **PhosChol.** Also add **Super Milk Thistle X** (1-2 caps, 2-3 times a day depending on the intensity of infection-fighting and liver-boosting you need). Not everyone gets overcome by these bugs, only those who need a nutrient boost. You have much more to choose from, depending on how much bug protection you need at the moment. As you correct your deficiencies you'll get stronger and need less.

Some of these items are so potent that they have been used to reverse old diseases as well as newer diseases like the recent onslaught of insulin resistance (a strong cardiovascular risk factor, also called metabolic syndrome X) and fatty liver diseases (that now affect one in five!) like **NASH** and **NAFLD** (<u>n</u>on-<u>a</u>lcoholic <u>s</u>teato<u>h</u>epatitis and <u>n</u>on-<u>a</u>lcoholic <u>f</u>atty <u>l</u>iver <u>d</u>isease) (Berkson, Buang, Oz, Arawal). Clearly the liver must be healthy to fight off infection. So how can you lose with so much to choose from?

Evidence:

- Linnanmaki E, et al, Chlamydia pneumoniae-specific circulating immune complexes in patients with chronic coronary heart disease, *Circulation,* 87:1130-4, 1993
- Saikku P, et al, Chronic **Chlamydia pneumoniae infection as a risk factor for coronary heart disease** in the Helsinki Heart Study, *Ann Intern Med,* 116:273-8, 1992
- Jackson LA, et al, Isolation of Chlamydia pneumoniae from a carotid endarterectomy specimen, *J Infect Dis,* 176:292-5, 1997
- Grayston JT, Infections caused by Chlamydia pneumoniae strain TWAR, *Clin Infect Dis,* 15:757-61, 1992
- Saikku P, et al, Serological evidence of an association of a novel chlamydia, TWAS, with chronic coronary heart disease and acute myocardial infarction, *Lancet,* 1988, ii: 983-986
- Muhlestin JB, et al, Increased Incidence of Chlamydia species within the coronary arteries of patients with symptomatic atherosclerotic versus other forms of cardiovascular disease, *J Am Coll Cardiol,* 27:1555-61, 1996
- Kusters JG, Kuipers EJ, **Helicobacter and atherosclerosis**, *Am Heart J,* 1999 Nov, 138(5 pt 2): S523-7
- Danesh J, et al, Is Helicobacter pylori a factor in coronary atherosclerosis? *J Clin Microbiol,* 1999 May, 37; 5:1651
- Sivam GP, et al, Helicobacter pylori – in vitro susceptibility to garlic (*Allium sativum*) extract, *Nutr Cancer,* 27; 2:118-21, 1997
- Berkson B, A conservative antioxidant approach to the treatment of hepatitis C. Combination of alpha lipoic acid (thioctic acid), silymarin and selenium: Three case histories, *Med Klin,* (Munich) 94;supple 3)84-9, 1999
- Agrawal S, et al, Management of nonalcoholic steatohepatitis: An analytic review, *J Clin Gastroenterol,* 35; 3:253-61, 2002

- Oz H, et al, **Glutathione-enhancing agents protect against steatohepatitis** in a dietary model, *J Biochem Mol Toxicol,* 20:2714-24, 2006
- Buang Y, et al, Dietary **phosphatidylcholine alleviates fatty liver** induced by orotic acid, *Nutr,* 21; 7-8:867-73, 2005
- Rogers SA, *No More Heartburn*, 2000, Kensington Publ NY and Prestige Publishing Syracuse NY (800-846-6687)
- Ruscin JM, et al, Vitamin B12 deficiency associated with histamine (2)-receptor antagonists and a proton-pump inhibitor, *Ann Pharmacother*, 36; 5:812-16, 2002
- Epstein M, et al, Proton-pump inhibitors and hypomagnesemic hypoparathyroidism, *N Engl J Med,* 355; 17:1834-6, 2006
- Ozutemiz AO, et al, Effect of omeprazole on plasma zinc levels after oral zinc administration, *Indian J Gastroenterol*, 21; 6:216-8, 2002

The Fibrinogen Clue

Clotting of blood is a major cause of heart attack. The higher your fibrinogen, a normal part of your clotting machinery, the more you are at risk (Yarnell). **One trigger of fibrinogen is chronic smoldering subclinical infection** (Patel). In fact, H. pylori and Chlamydia are associated with raised fibrinogen levels 66% and 80% of the time, respectively. *Helicobacter pylori* can be a silent infection of the stomach that is most often acquired in childhood and affects nearly half the adult population (Mendell). H. pylori, also causes raised fibrinogen levels since fostering chronic infection causes coronary clots.

Since **fibrinogen can also be a sign that a cancer is brewing or that the one you have is silently metastasizing or spreading**, you need to know a lot more about this, for which I refer you to more intensive reading *(TW)*. But nothing could be finer than to check the level now before you have nothing wrong with you or now if you already have problems. It helps you focus on the cause. If it is merely an infection that originates in the gut, see *No More Heartburn* for getting rid of it, and *The Cholesterol Hoax* for Chlamydia. And don't forget that **when any infection becomes resistant to treatment, most likely heavy metals are on board thwarting your efforts** (Summers). *The High Blood Pressure*

Hoax shows you in detail how to get rid of these. Never forget you may have to dig a lot deeper to uncover the clues for reversing your disease.

And before we leave this section on the buggy causes of heart disease, let me remind you once more that all the clues you learn about, regardless of case type, can help you later in your career as mystery-solver. For example, hidden nutrient deficiencies and toxicities like heavy metals or Teflon contribute not just to coronary artery disease, but to much other pathology from Alzheimer's to cancer. Likewise, these hidden bugs like H. pylori, can be the unsuspected cause of something as seemingly remote to you as **glaucoma** (Kountouras, also many highly referenced articles in *TW* for reversing "incurable" macular degeneration, etc.). Everything has a cause and a cure. We just happen to be focusing on the heart here. So why take eye drops the rest of your life and risk ultimate blindness when you might cure the problem?

Evidence:

- Kountouras J, et al, Eradication of *Helicobacter pylori* may be beneficial in the management of chronic open-angle glaucoma, *Arch Intern Med*, 162:1237-44, 2002
- Summers AO, et al, Genetic linkage of **mercury and antibiotic resistance in intestinal bacteria**, *Antimicrobial Agents Chemother*, 37:825-834,1993
- Patel P, et al, **Fibrinogen: a link between chronic infection and coronary heart disease**, *Lancet,* 343; 1634-5, June 25, 1994
- Yarnell JWG, et al, Fibrinogen, viscosity, and white blood cell count are major risk factors for ischaemic heart disease, *Circul,* 83:836-44, 1991
- Mendell MA, et al, Relation of *Helicobacter pylori* **infection and coronary heart disease**, *Brit Heart J,* 71:437-39, 1994

The Crime of Concealing the Evidence
For Slowing Down Coronary Calcifications

Once you know you have coronary calcifications, there are many things you need to do to slow down the progression. Your many choices are beyond the scope of this small treatise, but let's look at some simple ones. **Kyolic Liquid** is one proven exclusive proprietary formulation of aged garlic extract that has cut the progression of coronary calcifications by over a third with just a couple of squirts down the throat twice a day (Budoff). Likewise, anywhere from 1000-3000 mg of **Arginine Powder** twice a day has slowed progression of coronary calcifications (Boger), as have a variety of antioxidants (Hodis) and other nutrients. Arginine likewise can actually *cure* high blood pressure in lots of folks, and it even makes blood less able to form clots in folks who have high cholesterol (Wolf). And this information is over 10 years old in a high profile cardiology journal! See *The High Blood Pressure Hoax* for much more heart-saving that Arginine does.

In another study, 800 I.U. of **vitamin E a day dramatically cut the incidence of heart attack by over 70%**. With that kind of evidence, it seems unconscionable for insurance companies to deny coverage for not only vitamin E blood levels, but the nutrient itself, especially given the fact that they unquestionably cover drugs like Plavix®, proven to not be any better than aspirin but costing about $4 a capsule (details and references in *The Cholesterol Hoax)* (Davey, Winslow). Meanwhile as one more quick example out of many, **vitamins C and E slowed progression of arteriosclerosis in patients who even had heart transplants**. And these folks have a most dangerous scenario, for rarely if ever are their healing nutrients measured and corrected before or after such a nutrient-depleting procedure.

In a study by NIA, part of NIH, they followed 11,178 seniors, aged 67-105 for 9 years. Those who took **400 I.U. of vitamin E daily had a 41% reduction in heart disease, plus a 22% reduction in death from cancer and a 27% decrease in death overall from any cause** (Losonczy). Yet every cardiologist in the country does not recommend it. Why not? Sometimes the reason they use is that it could increase your bleeding time. But that is the very thing that they recommend folks take a daily aspirin for! Don't they see the contradiction here? On top of that, there is no drug that cuts heart disease 41%!

Evidence:

- Budoff MJ, et al, **Inhibiting progression of coronary calcifications using aged garlic extract** in patients receiving statin therapy: a preliminary study, *Preventive Medicin,e* 39; 5:985-91, 2004
- Siegel G, et al, Inhibition of arteriosclerotic plaque development by garlic, *Wien Med Wochenschr,* 154; 21-22:515-22, 2004
- Meema HE, et al, Serum magnesium level and arterial calcifications in end-stage renal disease, *Kidney Internat,* 32; 3:388-94, 1987
- Leonard F, et al, Initiation and inhibition of subcutaneous calcification, *Calc Tissue Res*, 10:269-79, 1972
- Boger RH, et al, Dietary **L-arginine reduces the progression of atheros-clerosis** in cholesterol-fed rabbits, *Circul,* 96:1282-90, 1997
- Hodis HN, Mack WJ, Azen SP, et al, Serial coronary angiographic evidence that **antioxidant vitamin intake reduces progression of coronary artery atherosclerosis**, *J American Med Assoc*, 1995; 273:1849-54
- Davey PJ, et al, Cost-effectiveness of vitamin E therapy in the treatment of patients with angiographically proven coronary narrowing (CHAOS) trial), Cambridge Heart Antioxidant Study, *Am J Cardiol,* 1998; 82:414-417
- Losonczy KG, et al, **Vitamin E and vitamin C supplement use and risk of all-cause and coronary heart disease mortality** in older persons: The established populations for epidemiologic studies of the elderly, *Amer J Clin Nutr,* 64; 2:190-6, Aug 1996
- Wolf A, et al, Dietary **arginine supplementation normalizes platelet ag-gregation** in hypercholesterolemic humans, *J Am Coll Cardiol*, 29:479-85, 1997
- Winslow R, et al, **Plavix® plus aspirin shows few benefits**, *Wall St J*, B3, Mar 13, 2006

The "K" Clue

What has your cardiologist recommended to you about vitamin K? Nothing? That's the norm. Ask any of them if you should be on it and see the response. It varies from "You don't want your blood to clot any faster. That's why I recommended aspirin and Plavix®" to "Absolutely not". "You are on Coumadin® to thin your blood and it would be counter-productive". Now let's show you the evidence and let you decide whether you should be on it and re-adjust your Coumadin® dose accordingly.

Coumadin®, the most commonly prescribed blood thinner, works by poisoning an enzyme essential in vitamin K chemistry (vitamin K epoxide reductase). This leads to serious damaging chemical changes in the body (Fiore). For starters, **Coumadin® fosters heart disease and osteoporosis, since it pulls calcium out of bone and dumps it into arteries**. And since Coumadin® lowers vitamin K, this puts folks at further risk for osteoporosis and joint replacements (Szulc, Shearer, Einhorn, Binkley). So expect to see (as we are) more osteoporosis, hip fractures, hip replacements, as well as unwanted calcifications in the arteries of the heart, heart valves, brain and legs, just as we do. In fact, lots of folks are silently deficient in vitamin K to begin with (unhealthy guts, past antibiotics, poor diet choices) leaving them with osteoporosis or these other maladies without even taking Coumadin®, as studies confirm. But once someone starts on Coumadin®, the damage is accelerated since **Coumadin® poisons vitamin K's action**. Of course these can all be measured and tailored to your body's needs, just as Coumadin® doses have been for decades.

You might think that you would know if you are low in vitamin K2, perhaps with easy bruising. But unfortunately **even a very mild or marginal vitamin K deficiency that produces no other symptoms can trigger calcification of arteries** (Jie). In medicine when someone has something like atrial fibrillation, cardiologists expect them to get worse as a natural course of events "because they are old". But it turns out that **Coumadin®** can be the cause, since **it accelerates arteriosclerosis or calcification of arteries and calcification of heart valves as well** (Vermeer, Price). For by inhibiting vitamin K action, Coumadin® (warfarin) pulls calcium out of the bones and dumps it into the coronary arteries and heart valves that eventually end up with surgery.

In one study of around 5,000 people, **vitamin K cut the calcifications of the aorta by 29%.** This is important because as the aorta calcifies it can lead to high blood pressure or heart failure, or form an aneurysm (the weakened wall balloons out). When the calcium cracks and the weakened arterial wall blows out, this rupture is usually lethal within minutes. Also when the aorta is calcified usually there is concomitant calcification of the coronary arteries leading to heart attacks, or calcification of heart valves leading to arrhythmias, extreme shortness of breath, ankle swelling, heart failure, and surgery or death. Furthermore, as the aorta becomes calcified this can also lead to intermittent claudication, manifested by severe pains and weakness in the legs with extended walking.

A major event as our heart and arteries age is they become stiff. What makes us lose elasticity? Elastin fiber. And what does elastin need? Lysyl oxidase (which needs copper), silicon (see source at end of this chapter and see more about it in *Pain Free In 6 Weeks*), enzymes (described in preceeding chapters, *TW, Wellness Against All Odds*), and vitamin K2 (Seyama).

Meanwhile, show your doctor the data in *The High Blood Pressure Hoax* and *Total Wellness* 2008 that you need 5 mg of Vitamin K2 a day for multiple reasons: (1) to counter the bone lose of Coumadin®, (2) to prevent unwanted calcification effects of Coumadin® in coronary arteries and heart valves, and (3) to reduce your rate of heart attack and slow down plaque progression (Geleijnse). Best of all, for folks who have already started "Kalcifying" their arteries, vitamin **K** actually can rip the "Kalcium" off the arterial wall, causing what we call **regression of plaque**. This is seriously important. There are no drugs that make coronary plaque melt away as well as nutrients do. And yes, **it is safe to take K with Coumadin®, as well as necessary** (show him the evidence in the books and have him adjust your dose).

Many **nutrients contribute to actual melting away (regression) of coronary plaque** or at the very least, dramatically slowing it down. These include for example, not only one **Vitamin K2** (menaquinone), but 1-2 a day of the best form of 2000 I.U. vitamin D3 (cholecaliciferol) that I know of, **Solar D Gems**, plus docosahexaenoic acid 500mg in one **Super DHA**, the eight forms of vitamin E in the form of 1-2 **E Gems Elite** plus 1 **Gamma E Gems** daily and 2 **Tocotrienol**s twice a day, not to mention enough magnesium that you learned about, and the oil change. There is much more that you haven't learned about yet, if you need it. Follow the directions for actually reversing and melting away coronary deposits in *The Cholesterol Hoax*. Your life depends on it.

Evidence:

- Geleijnse JM, et al, Dietary intake of **menaquinone is associated with a reduced risk of coronary heart disease**: The Rotterdam Study, *J Nutr,* 134: 3100-05, 2004
- Fiore CE, Tamburino C, Grimaldi D, et al, Reduced bone mineral content in patients taking an oral anticoagulant, *South Med J,* 83: 538-42, 1990
- Szulc P, Arlot M, Delmas PD, et al, Serum undercarboxylated osteocalcin is a marker of the risk of hip fracture in elderly women, *J Clin Invest,* 91: 769-74, 1993
- Shearer MJ, Vitamin K, *Lancet,* 345: 229-34, Jan. 28, 1995
- Einhorn TA, et al, Fracture healing and osteocalcin metabolism in vitamin K deficiency, *Clin Orthop,* 237:219-25, 1988
- Hodges SJ, et al, Circulating levels of vitamins K1 and K2 decreased in elderly women with hip fracture, *J Bone Miner Res,* 8; 10:1241-15, 1993
- Vermeer C, et al, Role of **K vitamins in the regulation of tissue calcification,** *J Bone Min Metab,* 19:201-06, 2001
- Spronk HMH, et al, Tissue-specific utilization **of menaquinone-4 results in prevention of arterial calcification in warfarin-treated** rats, *J Vasc Res,* 40:531-7, 2003
- Witteman JC, et al, Aortic calcification as a predictor of cardiovascular mortality, *Lancet,* 2:1120-22, 1986
- Binkley NC, et al, Vitamin K nutrition and osteoporosis, *J Nutr,* 125;7:1812-21, 1995
- Vermeer C, Schurfers LJ, A comprehensive review of vitamin K and vitamin K antagonist, *Blood Stasis & Thrombosis,* 14; 2: 339-53, April 2000
- Jie KSG, Bots ML, Grobbee DE, et al, Vitamin K status and bone mass in women with and without aortas with artherosclerosis: a population-based study, *Calcified Tissue Internat,* 59: 3 52-56, 1996
- Price PA, Faus SA, Williamson MK, **Warfarin causes rapid calcification of the elastic lamellae in rat arteries and heart valves,** *Arterioscler Thromb Vasc Biol,* 18:1400-07, 1998
- Seyama Y, Hayashi M, Usami E, et al, Comparative effects of vitamin K2 and vitamin E on experimental arteriosclerosis, *Internat J Vit Nutr Res,* 69; 1:23-26, 1999

- Seyama Y, et al, Atherosclerosis and matrix dystrophy, J *Atheroscleros Thromb*, 11: 236-45, 2004

Boost Nutrients In Order to Survive the Hospital

I keep hearing horror stories of how a relative went into the hospital for some elective surgical procedure and died. In this era it is to my way of thinking inexcusable to operate on anyone without knowing their nutrient status, and at least their anti-oxidant vitamins. For study after study confirms that those **who enter the hospital with the highest nutrient levels on board are the ones who survive**. Not only that, but they have fewer infections and other complications and get out of the hospital quicker, thus saving money and chance of complications. And for folks who end up in the hospital as an emergency, even those who are **the most sick and in danger of dying at any moment in the intensive care unit** (as from overwhelming infection called sepsis), **nutrients have been the only thing that has rescued them and chopped the death rate in half**.

As I explained and referenced in much more detail in *The High Blood Pressure Hoax*, folks who were in ICU near death, when medicine had nothing else to offer, were given something outrageous as a desperate last resort: **Vitamin C (500 mg) and Vitamin E (400 IU).** There was (for those lucky enough to get the nutrients) a **57% increase in survival in the folks who got pennies worth of nutrients in ICU.** But do you know of a hospital that carries these in its pharmacy? Have you ever seen the look on a cardiologist's face when you ask for these? He is so incredulous that you would think you had just dropped your drawers in front of him.

And you need only glance through a few weeks of *The Wall Street Journal* to be convinced of the fact that being in the hospital is one of the most dangerous places anywhere, since it contains the highest number of antibiotic-resistant bugs, not to mention a concentration of medical errors.

If you have the option to schedule a hospital admission in advance, I would definitely recommend getting your nutrients in the best shape possible. You can use the programs in the books, and be sure to do the oil change and mineral replacement as a bare minimum, as outlined in *The Cholesterol Hoax*. Optimum is to get a **Cardio/ION Panel** that then spells out your particular nutrient deficiencies. Plus it goes one step further accomplishing something that no other available test can do. It actually shows you and your doctor your individual requirements for certain nutrients that may be above and beyond the standard recommended daily allowance (RDA). You may need more than "normal".

Evidence:

- Porter JM, Ivatury RR, Azimuddin K, et al, Antioxidant therapy in the prevention of organ dysfunction syndrome and infectious **complications after trauma**: early results of a prospective randomized study, *Am Surg,* 65: 4 78-4 83, 1999
- Cowley HC, Bacon OJ, Goode HF, et al, Plasma antioxidant potential in **severe sepsis**: a comparison of survivors and nonsurvivors, *Crit Care Med,* 24: 1179-83, 1996
- Nathens AB, Neff MJ, Jurkovich GJ, et al. Randomized, prospective trial of antioxidant supplementation in **critically ill surgical patients**, *Ann Surgery,* 236: 8 14-8 22, 2002

Does "D" Stand for Double Jeopardy Or "Don't Double Your Chance to Die" Early?

I know when you think of vitamin D you probably think of bones and teeth. But having a **low level of vitamin D actually doubles your chance of an early heart attack and is more predictive of early death than a high cholesterol level.** Furthermore there is a hidden epidemic of vitamin D deficiency in the United States, the land of plenty. Harvard University's School of Public Health studied over 18,000 male health professionals for over 10 years. They found that a low or even "normal" level of vitamin D is a strong risk factor for early heart disease, doubling the chance of an early heart attack.

Some unknowledgeable docs have even warned their patients that a higher amount of vitamin D could add to calcification of their coronary arteries. On the contrary, **the higher the vitamin D level, the lower the coronary calcifications.** And this is right out of a major cardiology journal over a decade ago. Why didn't this make news? And who reads this stuff? Certainly not your average cardiologist, or he would be checking your level of vitamin D routinely. In fact **vitamin D makes arteries more stable and less likely to rupture**. Use the protocols in *The Cholesterol Hoax* to reverse or at least slow down coronary plaque.

And this doesn't even count the unnecessary deaths from other aspects of vitamin D deficiency. For a level of vitamin D inadequate for your body raises the incidence of hypertension and diabetes (two very serious cardiovascular risk factors), as well and as cancers, infections, multiple sclerosis, and more. Between sunscreens, cloudy weather, northern climates, and sitting at computers most of the time, most folks do not get enough sun to make sufficient vitamin D in their bodies. Add to this the fact that phthalates or plasticizers damage the chemistry of cholesterol and other chemistry involved in processing vitamin D in the body, it becomes clear that we all need to supplement. I can vouch for that, especially after seeing the low levels in "healthy" folks in Florida who have taken nutrients for years and who get plenty of sunshine.

Make sure you take at least one **Solar D Gems 2000 mg** a day, then check your level to be sure it is at least higher than the minimum 30 ng/ml (or 65 nmol/L, depending on the units of measure the lab uses). Studies prove it really is best to be above 60 ng/ml. Be careful to see your lab results, since some labs still use the old antiquated cut-off for "normal" that is much lower.

Evidence:

- Giovannucci E, Liu Y, Hollis BW, et al, 25-**hydroxyvitamin D and risk of myocardial infarction** in men, *Arch Intern Med,* 168:1174-80, 2008
- Watson KE, et al, Active serum **vitamin D levels are inversely correlated with coronary calcification,** *Circulation,* 96; 6:1755-60, 1997
- Dobnig H, Independent association of low serum 25-hydroxyvitamin D and 1,25-dihydroxyvitamin D levels with all-cause and cardiovascular mortality, *Arch Intern Med,* 168; 12:1340-49, 2008
- Milma U, et al, **Vitamin D supplementation reduces cardiovascular events** in a subgroup of middle-aged individuals with both type 2 diabetes mellitus and the haptoglobin 2-2 genotype. A prospective double-blinded clinical trial, *Arterioscl Thromb Vasc Biol,* v28, 2008

Diffusing the D-Defense

Important repeat: Is your doctor using the commonly accepted "norm" that is antiquated and proven to be screamingly inferior? Please don't let him settle for anything less than 65 nmol/L (30 ng/ml, but aim for 60). For if your lab value is in the middle of the "normal" range, where the majority of the population falls, you have more than doubled your chances of an early heart attack and other chronic diseases. If seeing you in the top quintile or above scares him off, have him catch up on *TW* 2008 (and he might actually read the references here and in *The Cholesterol Hoax*).

If you have coronary calcifications on your ultra fast heart scan, do you think this is a guaranteed determinant of early cardiac death? On the flip side, if your heart scan (or angiography) is negative, do you think your chances of sudden cardiac arrest are slim? Wrong on both accounts if you answered, "Yes".

I want to make it clear. The **chances of early heart death, regardless of what your coronary heart scan shows are more than triply tied to the level of one nutrient, vitamin D**. In fact, **the chance for early death is even higher in folks without coronary calcifications than those with calcifications - - - - if they are in the "normal" range for vitamin D**. For the "normal" range is now proven to be too low. In **fact if you are in the "normal" range for vitamin D, it places you in the category of having triple risk of early heart attack, regardless of your coronary calcium score.**

Meanwhile, if you are low, you may need as much as 1-2 **Solar D Gems** 2000 IU daily, depending on where you are starting from, your personal load of toxins, and other parameters on your **Cardio/ION** results. **A respectable level of vitamin D triples your chance of staving off an early heart attack as well as cuts your risk of diabetes in half, lowers your propensity for falls and accidents, infections, high blood pressure, high triglycerides, accelerated ageing, osteoporosis, cancer, MS, depression, allergies**, and much more. Sorry for the repetition (no I'm not), but this is absolutely crucial to your survival!

And remember, I stressed vitamin D in this section to give you an example of the overwhelmingly important relation of merely one vitamin that hardly any cardiologist ever checks. This is in spite of a mountain of evidence proving it is staggeringly important to his specialty. You deserve a cardiologist who is focused on keeping you alive and healthy and drug-free. Many other nutrients share the scene in importance.

Will Vitamin D Calcify Coronary Arteries?

No. In fact just the opposite is true. It's true that the calcification in coronary artery plaque looks similar to the formation of bone. And certainly unwanted calcium in the heart valves and arteries is a major cause of heart surgery death in this country. In fact vascular calcification is so widespread that over 90% of patients with coronary heart disease have calcifications somewhere else in the body's vascular tree.

Vitamin D is actually needed to lower the amount of vascular calcification and keep calcium in the bones where it belongs

and not dumped into the arteries and heart valves where it doesn't belong. Furthermore, there is a significant association of osteoporosis in patients with the vascular calcifications. When nutrient deficiencies, toxic levels of heavy metals and other chemicals, or kidney disease (from heavy metals) as examples, interfere with proper bone growth, the calcium is dumped into the toxic waste site, which are the arteries and heart valves.

Further research shows that vitamin D3 (cholecaliciferol, not the cheaper synthetic D2!) deficiency makes the heart more irritable, thus promoting arrhythmias and makes the heart muscle cells enlarge and become fibrotic (like scar tissue, without much blood supply or muscle action) as in congestive heart failure and cardiomyopathies and myocarditis. **Vitamin D deficiency is clearly a risk for heart disease, plus its deficiency is epidemic.**

You may not know that vitamin D requires normal cholesterol metabolism. But recall that **statin drugs poison cholesterol chemistry.** Plus the **plasticizers (phthalates) poison cholesterol metabolism** (through beta-oxidation), while **heavy metals damage the kidneys** where further vitamin D metabolism occurs. And clearly all the vitamin D in the world won't help if the vitamin D receptors in cell membranes are not healthy. That's where the oil change, as described earlier, comes in. See how all this ties in? No wonder many researchers have shown that **a low vitamin D presents even a higher risk for early coronary artery disease than having an elevated coronary calcium score.**   And that was over a decade ago in a major cardiology journal, ostensibly read by the cardiology community. O.K., I promise, that's all on D.

Evidence:
- Watson KE, et al, Active **serum vitamin D levels are inversely correlated with coronary calcifications,** *Circulation,* 96:1755-60, 1997
- Rahman A, et al, Heart extracellular matrix gene expression profile in the vitamin D receptor knockout mice, *J Steroid Biochem Molec Biol,* 103:416-19, 2007

- Dobnig H, et al, Independent association of low serum 25-hydroxy vitamin D and 1, 25-dihydroxyvitamin D levels with all-cause and cardiovascular mortality, *Arch Intern Med,* 168; 12:1340-49, 2008

Can He Be Guilty of Ignorance?

Why hasn't the field of cardiology taught folks how to slow down and even reverse calcifications? Ask most cardiologists and see what kind of answer you get. Fortunately you now know vitamin D puts calcium in the bones where it belongs, and keeps it out of the arteries. In fact folks with higher levels of D have half the heart death of those at the lower end of "normal". Likewise, **vitamin K** (menaquinone) is another crucial nutrient that **cuts calcification of the aorta (the main artery from the heart) in half** (Geleijnse). But why don't cardiologists know this stuff? Is there any excuse for this when much of the information has been in their leading journals for years? Why haven't they as leaders in cardiovascular health been at least measuring these, much less prescribing them? Is this negligence? Ignorance? Laziness? I don't know.

That's one more reason why I think it's imperative for anyone wanting to not only decrease heart disease but all other types of diseases to at least have daily 1 each **Solar D Gems** and **Vitamin K2**. For calcification of arteries leads to poorer nutrient delivery to that organ and eventual premature death of that organ. Plus, as always with the nutritional approach to medical treatment, there are multiple benefits. These are among the same nutrients critical for preventing and/or curing osteoporosis. And they are needed for strong ligaments and tendons and blood vessels. Both of these nutrients are easily measured with your **Cardio/ION**. When was the last time you had your vitamins D and K measured?

And don't forget this is just the tip of the iceberg of what makes plaque not only slow down, but also regress and melt away. Phosphatidylcholine is one more of these (Stafford), one more reason why daily **PhosChol** is crucial (see *The Cholesterol Hoax* for the many nutrients and easy tests needed for regression (melting away) of plaque and directions, sources, etc.).

Evidence:
- Stafford WW, et al, **Regression of atherosclerosis** affected by intravenous phospholipid, *Artery*, 1:106-114, 1975
- Watson KE, et al, Active serum **vitamin D levels are inversely correlated with coronary calcifications,** *Circulation,* 96:1755-60, 1997
- Geleijnse JM, et al, Dietary intake of **menaquinone is associated with a reduced risk of coronary heart disease**: The Rotterdam Study, *J Nutr,* 134: 3100-05, 2004
- Rogers SA, *The High Blood Pressure Hoax*, prestigepublishing.com
- Rogers, SA, *The Cholesterol Hoax*, prestigepublishing.com

Is Withholding Information Criminal?

Once you have been rescued from the jaws of death through heroic measures of cardiologists, it is natural to be grateful and awed by their expertise. But realize that you cannot afford to assume that just because they are terrific at the emergent part, that this trans-lates automatically to the hereafter. Now is the time to go for the biochemical cause, correction and cure. Ask your cardiologist how he plans to assay and correct your levels of vitamin D, alpha and gamma tocopherol, K, and fatty acids, especially EPA, DHA, GLA, and trans fats, plus minerals like RBC magnesium, selenium, chromium, manganese, and copper, plus amino acids like arginine, taurine, and more.

The point of this is to show you that you have so much more con-trol over your destiny than you have ever been led to believe. And once you have had a cardiac diagnosis (like calcified coronary ar-teries or valves), or a cardiac event (like a heart attack) or surgic-al intervention (like stents or bypass or ablation), your knowledge becomes even more crucial to your survival. Yet many times the authorities whose hands you place your life in have either not bo-thered to learn this or have withheld the information in here that is so critical to your longevity.

Solution Sources

For folks who would like one easy source for all of their nutrients in this book, **NEEDS** carries them (needs.com or 1-800-634-1380).

Item	Web/Company	800#
Solar D Gems, Vitamin K2	carlsonlabs.com	323-4141
Super DHA, Arginine Powder	carlsonlabs.com	323-4141
E Gems Elite, Gamma E Gems	carlsonlabs.com	323-4141
Tocotrienols, Cod Liver Oil, Fish Oil	carlsonlabs.com	323-4141
Cardio/ION	metametrix.com	221-4640
Kyolic Liquid	kyolic.com	421-2998
NSC-24 Beta Glucan Circulatory Formula,	nsc 24.com	888-541-3997
SeaSel	intensivenutrition.com	333-4141
PhosChol	nutrasal.com	777-1886
Super Milk Thistle X	integrativeinc.com	931-1709

Chapter VI

Solving the Crime

Are You a Model Patient?

In 2008 there was scarcely an American who wasn't saddened and surprised by the untimely death of NBC commentator, host of *Meet the Press,* and longtime political interviewer revered for his fairness and lack of bias. But his death taught us more than he ever dreamed of in life. Hundreds of internet sites and many TV interviews attacked the question: How did a man who was described by his own doctor as a "model patient" die of a sudden heart attack at his desk, and die from his first one, at the tender age of 58? It is hard to know exactly all of the ramifications, having not been his physician, but there are some lessons to be learned perhaps.

Numerous newspaper and magazine articles as well as internet sites reported that he was on all the classic medications prescribed by cardiologists in 2008: a statin for his cholesterol, Plavix® and an aspirin to stop clots and heart attacks, and a blood pressure medicine. He had calcification of his LAD (left anterior descending) coronary artery, with a calcium score of 210 in 1998. He also had mild hypertension, elevated triglycerides (for which he took a diabetes medication), all controlled. He used an exercise bike and took his medicines.

His most recent blood work showed a cholesterol of a staggering 105 and a rock bottom low HDL of 37. Not only was a statin drug perhaps inappropriate for this man, but aside from too low a cholesterol (you need at least a 200 to make hormones, and repair brain, heart and other tissues), it also poisoned his liver enzyme (HMG CoA reductase) that makes CoQ10. This CoQ10 deficiency leads then to heart failure. So not surprisingly on autopsy he had an enlarged heart, the early stage of heart failure.

In addition, poisoning the enzyme to make cholesterol leads to high blood pressure by compromising the beta-receptors and calcium channels in heart cell membranes. As a consequence, beta-blockers and calcium channel blockers are popularly used for the resultant hypertension. But beta-blockers for high blood pressure raise triglycerides and diabetes, lower CoQ10 and zinc, and lower HDL. Since this is the exact opposite of what you want, both of these propel you toward a faster death.

But the damage is just beginning once you start another drug. For example, beta-blockers (prescribed for high blood pressure, stage fright, arrhythmias and more) kill your thyroid gland function bringing on weight that won't budge, exhaustion, depression, hair and tooth loss, not to mention heart failure and more. They also lower zinc needed to stave off cancer, heart disease plus more. You see **every drug catapults you into a myriad of other illnesses**. But by all modern standards, this broadcasting icon had the standard of care rendered by United States cardiologists. In addition to this, there are a multitude of other reasons why he prematurely died. So let's see how his legacy can keep you from going down that road.

Early Warnings

- **Half the people who have their first heart attack die from it.** They never get a chance to have bypass or a stent or medical management, and have no warning. And half never had high cholesterol.
- **Statins do not lower the overall death rate**. Half the folks on statin cholesterol-lowering drugs go on to have a heart attack anyway. Statins do not guarantee safety.
- Plavix® was shown at the American College of Cardiology meeting to be no better than aspirin at protecting folks. And aspirin has finally been shown to be without benefit. Yet Plavix®, laden with undesirable side effects, is heavily prescribed in spite of this evidence. Plus **being concomitantly on a sta-**

tin negates the benefit of expensive Plavix®. The one drug actually cancels out the benefit of the other, but still many cardiologists prescribe the two.

- **Aspirin does not protect against a heart attack**, and in fact doubles the risk of stroke. But it remains common advise by the majority of cardiologists who are led by pharmaceutical hype versus biochemical facts. They have failed to learn about the nutrients that are far better at protecting the heart (all detailed between the *Total Wellness* newsletter, *The Cholesterol Hoax,* and *The High Blood Pressure Hoax*, complete with scientific backup for all doctors).

- **Cholesterol of 105 is dangerously low** and deprives the heart of one of the very nutrients it needs to repair and survive, plus it leads to suicidal depression, as the brain is starved as well.

- The torturous **low cholesterol diet is not necessary and in fact is harmful.** The liver makes cholesterol every day. Once you have "fixed" your broken chemistry that created high cholesterol or heart disease (even disease without any cholesterol problem), you can eat the cholesterol goodies you want. The healthy body balances it out.

But more importantly, there are **tests that are commonly ignored by the majority of cardiologists that are over four times more powerful than cholesterol in predicting an early heart attack**. And the beauty of knowing this chemistry is that **all these tests are reversible and correctable**. It **is like having your own personal crystal ball**. Unfortunately most cardiologists are not aware of these tests and this is in spite of the fact that the enormous amount of scientific backup for them is from their very own journals.

Why are homocysteine, fibrinogen, insulin, hsCRP, RBC magnesium, RBC zinc, vitamin D, vitamin K, eicosapentaenoic acid (EPA), docosahexanenoic acid (DHA), kynurenate, beta-hydroxyisovalerate, testosterone and many other tests not routinely done? Of course for hormone deficiencies there are drugs, but even then the solution should not be to take a hormone (which turns off gland function through feedback inhibition). But rather the goal should be to repair and detoxify the damaged hormone pathway. Lots of folks, for example have gotten off thyroid medication, even though they were told they would need it for life, once they detoxified their thyroids (see *Detoxify or Die* for starters).

These crystal ball danger indicators (and many more) are all corrected with non-prescription nutrients. Even a most recent medical warning has once more confirmed that we can (1) cut the chance of dying of a heart attack by more than half, (2) reduce heart enlargement, (3) plus lower triglycerides, (4) lower blood pressure, and (5) raise HDL, (6) plus reduce the chance of ventricular fibrillation just by taking DHA (docosahexanenoic acid), a part of cod liver oil. I recommend one **Super DHA** a day.

But don't forget that for this simple and inexpensive item, DHA, to work, you must get the plastics out of your system, because they poison the carnitine, which in turn is needed to allow the healing fatty acid, DHA, to replace the bad ones (*Detoxify or Die* explains that).

Vitamins K2, D3, EPA, DHA, phosphatidyl choline, gamma tocopherol, plus DHA and many other nutrients are crucial in slowing down the progression of coronary calcifications and even more important **in reversing coronary calcifications**. But it all hinges on the doctor knowing all the facts and directions spelled out in *The Cholesterol Hoax*. That is precisely why I took enormous time out of my life to write it for you. For if we wait for medicine to catch up, if we wait for every cardiologist to learn and apply these tools to save lives, it may not realistically come in our lifetimes.

Where Has 30 Years of Progress Led Us?

The sad fact is that even if you are famous, even if you are a millionaire, **you cannot buy health. You cannot afford to leave it**

to the "specialists" who are unknowingly controlled by the pharmaceutical industry. You must take the bull by the horns and learn how to save yourself. Want to know another discouraging fact?

My father, a hard-working man who never graduated from high school, raised 8 children and never had the time or money to go to a doctor, never took medicines, ate the wrong foods, and smoked 2 packs daily of unfiltered cigarettes for over 40 years. And he had familial high cholesterol, the worst kind. He died at the same age as our 2008-broadcasting icon, 58, of a sudden heart attack, but 32 years ago. Does this remind you of the American Cancer Society data I have given in *TW* in the past? Recall that they showed that with all the billions of dollars given to them, the overall improvement in survival for cancer in the last 30 years is 0.7%, less than 1% !!!

Where did all the high tech medicine, time and money spent over the last 3 decades go? My father had no money, no doctor, no medications, a worse family history (all generations of men died before 58), plus more than 5 major coronary arteries blocked on autopsy and high cholesterol, in addition to his high stress load (me as a daughter, for one), bad diet, and 2 packs of unfiltered Lucky Strikes® a day for 32 years. The TV broadcasting icon, on the other hand, (1) had the benefit of modern medicine 32 years later after many more advances in medicine had been made, (2) he was a millionaire, (3) he was on all the expensive medications prescribed, (4) he did not smoke, (5) he had only one vessel damaged with plaque, and (6) he was described as a "model patient" by his doctor.

No, I believe that you will agree with me once you read the evidence, that the current cardiology practice is more favorable to the bottom line of the pharmaceutical companies than it is to your bottom line of healthy longevity. The evidence in *The Cholesterol Hoax* will convince you, as it should since it is right out of the leading cardiology journals, of what you have to do to save your life and the lives of those you love. For even if you don't have high cholesterol or are too young to be even concerned about it, remember that **half the people who die of a sudden heart attack never even had high cholesterol, but they did have the risk factors, all of which are correctable** and described in the book.

And the age of death is getting startlingly lower. Furthermore, for the healthy person, the protocols in the book constitute **the best anti-aging armamentarium I know of, for it spells out what nutrients are most commonly low in the majority of folks who are assayed with the crystal ball test.** This is especially important if you cannot afford to do the test. As well, it contains what you need to know to stave off Alzheimer's, Parkinson's, cancers, and other end-stages of body deterioration, called chronic diseases by pharmacy-focused medicine.

What should you do today? Get your cardiologist to order the best crystal ball test I know of, the **Cardio/ION**, to highlight your hidden deficiencies and toxicities that have created your disease, or that will create disease and accelerate ageing in your future if you don't reverse them now. If you need help, I have scheduled personal phone consultations with our readers (dedicated and thorough, please) to assist their doctors in interpreting their possibilities.

Evidence:
- Siddiqui RA, et al, Modulation of enzymatic activities by n-3 polyunsaturated fatty acids to support cardiovascular health, *J Nutr Biochem,* 19:417-37, 2008
- Castillo A, et al, Docosahexaenoic acid inhibits protein kinase C translocation/activation and cardiac hypertrophy in rat cardiomyocytes, *J Mol Genet Med,* 1:18-25, 2005
- Takahashi R, et al, Dietary fish oil attenuates cardiac hypertrophy in lipotoxic cardiomyopathy due to systemic carnitine deficiency, *Cardiovasc Res*, 68:213-23, 2005
- Yin K, et al, Blood pressure and vascular reactivity changes in spontaneously hypertensive rats fed fish oil, *Br J Pharmacol,* 102:991-7, 1991

- Billman GE, et al, Prevention of ischemia-induced ventricular fibrillation by omega-3 fatty acids, *Proc Natl Acad Sci USA*, 91:4427-30, 1994
- Leaf A, Omega-3 fatty acids and prevention of ventricular fibrillation, *Prostaglandins Leukot Essent Fatty Acids*, 52:197-8, 1995
- Hallaq H, et al, Modulation of dihydropyridine-sensitive calcium channels in heart cells by fish oil fatty acids, *Prod Natl Acad Sci USA,* 89:1760-4, 1992
- McKenny JM, et al, Prescription of omega-3 fatty acids for the treatment of hypertriglyceridemia, *Am J Health Syst Pharm,* 64:595-605, 2007
- Theis F, et al, Association of n-3 polyunsaturated fatty acids with stability of atherosclerotic plaques: a randomized controlled trial, *Lancet,* 361:47-85, 2003
- Gruppo Italiano per lo Studio della Soprevvivenza nell'Infarto miocardico, Dietary supplementation with n-3 polyunsaturated fatty acids and vitamin E after myocardial infarction: results of the GISSI-Prevenzione trial, *Lancet,* 354:447-55, 1999

How About an Easy Start?

I know, you are overwhelmed and it seems like a daunting task. I agree. But every journey begins with one step. For those of you who are brand new to the concept that you have anything to do with whether or not you die of heart disease, and how soon that happens, welcome to the first day of the rest of your life. I know many of you feel overwhelmed, but don't be discouraged. All good and worthwhile things for which there is no substitute, whether building health or friendships, occurs in small bites or increments. So let's see something very simple that you could do today to start to turn the tide.

To make you feel more comfortable, let's take something right out of the high-profile *Journal of the American Medical Association* in the fall of 2006. Did you know just consuming **3-4 cups of green tea a day could cut your chance of dying of heart disease by more than a third** (Kuriyama)? Now how easy can that be? And why didn't this make the news like the studies full of flaws that attempted to denigrate nutrients? Because there's no money in drinking green tea.

My favorite source is **Sencha Premium Organic Green Tea** (available from indigo-tea.com). You merely put the loose tea leaves (free from dioxin-containing tea bags) into your **infuser** (available from natural-lifestyle.com) and steep with filtered hot water. What could be easier, more healthful and comforting all at once? It is a morning habit worth cultivating.

If you read further in the recommended books, you will learn that for the more serious cases and for healthy longevity, we all need to detoxify daily. Each night when we turn in, we have the chance right then to make our bodies better, same or worse. Those are the only directions we can go in. It is clear that **all heart disease suffers from insufficient detoxification**. Vitamin C, lipoic acid and glutathione are a powerful combo that jump-start detoxification, plus healing the cardiovascular diseases depend on these nutrients heavily (*Detoxify or Die* has a huge amount of references). What better time to do it than before bed when your body will be in its healing phase and repair mode?

Although our detox cocktail's ingredients are spelled out in higher doses and with more additions, there is a super easy start (and better tasting!). The **Daily Detox Drink** (happybodies.com) comes in easy travel packets or as a powder to mix any time with purified water. It is incredibly easy and great for beginners. And you need it whether you are healthy or have the worst heart disease…in fact any disease (Prasad, Krundieck, Packer, Rath,). And as the references show, its ingredients even reverse brain aging (Hagen, Liu). Furthermore, when someone has a heart attack, the levels of these nutrients take a nosedive even further (Usal). Remember, the same pathology happens in other organs, not just the heart. The best news is when you heal one organ you often heal another.

Evidence:
* Hagen TM, et al, R-Lipoic acid-supplemented old rats have **improved mitochondrial function**, decreased oxidative damage, and increased metabolic rate, *FASEB J*, 13:411-18, 19999

138

- Liu J, et al, **Memory loss** in old rats associated with brain mitochondrial decay and RNA/DNA oxidation: Partial **reversal** by feeding acetyl-L-carnitine and /or R-a-lipoic acid, *Proc Natl Acad Sci USA*, 99; 4:2356-61, 2002
- Usal A, et al, Decreased glutathione levels in acute myocardial infarction, *Jpn Heart J*, 37:177-82, 1996
- Prasad A, et al, Glutathione reverses endothelial dysfunction and improves nitric oxide bioavailability, *J Am Cardiol*, 34:5-7-14, 1999
- Rath M, Pauling L, Hypothesis: lipoprotein(a) is a surrogate for ascorbate, *Proc Natl Acad Sci USA*, 87:6204-7, 1990
- Kuriyama S, et al, **Green tea consumption and mortality due to cardiovascular disease, cancer, and all causes** in Japan, The Ohsaki Study, *J Am Med Assoc*, 296:1255-65, 2006
- Meister A, Glutathione-ascorbic acid antioxidant system in animals, *J Biolog Chem*, 269:9397-9400, 1994

For the More Advanced

On the flip side, from the same high profile journal, *JAMA*, we learned something more difficult to do. A modified macrobiotic diet can reverse heart disease symptoms and medicines in cases where medications are powerless. But to us this comes as no surprise, since for decades we have watched folks do the same when they were given mere days to live, bed-ridden with wildly metastatic cancer, inoperable, refractory to anything the oncologists had to offer. Yet the diet has reversed them and many are 10-20 years later and still very healthy. You don't hear about these documented cures, either, because there is no money in well people who have learned they don't need drugs, except for emergencies. In fact if you check out the American Cancer Society, they will advise against the macrobiotic diet (with no evidence to support their advice!).

If you need serious healing, the macrobiotic diet is enormously healing. I have personally seen it literally wipe out everything from allergies and rheumatoid arthritis to end-stage heart failure and cancer. To do it, read these in this order: *You Are What You Ate*, then *The Cure Is In the Kitchen*, and then *Macro Mellow*. Yet even then, if someone emergently has to address something serious like a cancer, but has not yet caught up in knowledge, start with the infinitely simpler *Wellness Against All Odds*. You can be dumb as a rock and learn how to juice carrots and do the detox enema and enzymes, as examples.

By the way, as my gift to you readers, feel free to get a free sample issue of my December 2006 *TW* newsletter that details how folks have kicked death in the teeth when given mere days to live by their doctors and told "There is nothing more that can be done". I hope you never fall for that line again. I hope you have learned that not only do you have enormous power over your cardiovascular system, but that you have been able to see how all this also applies to any disease, including the dreaded cancer.

By now many of you have realized that **disease names are merely labels with very little meaning. What matters most is what caused your symptoms**. For once you know the cause, you know how to cure it. For example, arrhythmias have lots more causes than I presented here. Sensitivities to foods, chemicals, molds, deficiencies of minerals, vitamins, fatty acids, amino acids, hormones, and more are common triggers. For more details, read *Depression Cured At Last!* For every item that can trigger brain dysfunction can also trigger cardiac arrhythmias as an example. The difference is merely the individual's target organ. This will give you a broader scope of knowledge about the vast possibilities of causes. The beauty is they are all correctable. And the beauty of healing naturally is that every organ benefits. Whereas **with pharmacy-focused medicine, every organ becomes the potential target for a dangerous side effect**. That is why there is a litany of symptoms described for every target organ in the book of abbreviated side effects, the *PDR (Physician's Desk Reference)*.

I have to handcuff myself to stop from giving you much more examples of empowerment, because I promised many I would make this a *short* book on evidence. For many folks are intimidated or scared off by a larger book. They go to their graves never realizing they had power over their health. But now that you understand how much power you have, you can then tackle the rest of the books that have the needed details. The neat thing about knowledge is that once it is given, it is yours forever. No one can take it away from you, it doesn't rust or rot, and it merely accumulates and grows into an increasingly useful tool. This book merely serves as a stepping-stone for further unbridled growth. If I included all the data contained in the other books, you would need a wheelbarrow to carry this book to the beach. The bottom line is that regardless of what type of non-cardiac labels you have been given, there is likewise a cause and a cure. This book merely uses the heart as the exemplary target organ.

Evidence:

- Ornish D, Intensive lifestyle changes for reversal of coronary heart disease, *J Amer Med Assoc,* 280:2001-2007, 1998
- Rogers SA, *You Are What You Ate*, prestigepublishing.com or 1-800-846-6687
- Rogers SA, *The Cure Is In the Kitchen*, prestigepublishing.com or 1-800-846-6687
- Rogers SA, *Macro Mellow*, prestigepublishing.com or 1-800-846-6687
- Rogers SA, *Wellness Against All Odds*, prestigepublishing.com or 1-800-846-6687
- Rogers SA, *Total Wellness* (newsletter), prestigepublishing.com or 1-800-846-6687

The Suspect Everybody Missed

There is one major cause of epidemic death that every one misses in all this. Even the medical folks miss it that label their practices the trendy terms like "functional medicine", "integrative medicine", environmental medicine, holistic medicine, "comprehensive", "anti-aging", and more. I have been to their meetings and even lectured there myself, heard the tapes and CDs from meetings I didn't attend, read the syllabi, voluminous journal articles, and more. It is universally absent.

There is one factor that contributes to more damaged human chemistry than all the others put together.

• You recall how important the fatty acids are in actually healing the heart. Well this factor poisons zinc so that the enzymes D-6-D (delta-6-desaturase) and D-5-D that convert fatty acids to their healing forms are paralyzed.

• You recall how a high homocysteine is 4 times more powerful a predictor of early death than a high cholesterol. Well this factor inhibits B6 conversion so that homocysteine goes up, triggering also Alzheimer's, blindness from macular degeneration, and eventually a litany of maladies.

This mystery factor damages every aspect of metabolism, poisoning your ability to heal. As a few more examples:

• It poisons B-oxidation of fatty acids so crucial for heart, blood vessel and nerve membranes.

• And even creates high cholesterol.

• It poisons the folic acid receptors on cell membranes, which then leads to increased heart disease, homocysteine elevations, cancer, Alzheimer's, and more.

• It poisons carnitine, needed to move the fatty acids into the cardiac mitochondria so energy can be produced.

• It poisons sulfation pathways so you can't detoxify environmental chemicals like diesel that trigger heart attacks and arrhythmias or even your own hormones.

• It creates a silent epidemic of malfunctioning thyroid glands (another cardiovascular risk factor).

• And is a major player in creating the epidemic of increased diabetes so bad that 1 in 8 children have what we used to call "adult onset diabetes".

• It can damage every gland.

• It creates insulin-resistance and metabolic syndrome and low testosterone, all of which trigger early heart death.

- It triggers not only heart problems in mature adults, but also heart problems in progressively younger adults. Dying of a sudden heart attack at 39 is no longer rare.
- And this mystery factor has contributed to a silent epidemic of cancers, from prostate to breast and more. Forty years ago when I was in medical school, cancer was rare and you never heard of it in kids. Now cancer is the number one cause of death in children 1-15 and young adults 25-45.
- Plus this mystery factor makes cancers medication-resistant.
- And **we cannot escape this factor tanking up in our bodies**.
- Because even the polar bears in the pristine Arctic have measurable levels. As a consequence, they also now have human diseases like hypothyroidism and osteoporosis. And even newborn babies have measurable levels of this mystery factor.

The mystery factor is **phthalates, the name for chemicals that outgas from plastics**. They permeate every aspect of life from our foods, water and air, from plastic beverage containers, cosmetics, and clothes to furnishings, construction materials, industrial and vehicular exhausts, computers, appliances, home wiring (it heats and outgases), medications, and a multitude of other sources. We cannot live without them nor escape them. They have permeated our lives. And low doses are more damaging than high.

And the American Plastics Council argues that they are safe, based on 11 studies done a quarter of a century ago. But prominent scientists around the world have proven with over 105 studies done with more modern technology that they can cause just about every abnormality in the body that we call disease. And why shouldn't they be a major player since their levels are over **10,000 times higher than any other human pollutant in the human body**. And **low doses are more dangerous than high**! We are the first generation of man to ever be living with so many chemicals in our bodies that axe normal chemistry in a myriad of ways.

The bad news? Phthalates, ubiquitously unavoidable, kill mitochondria, the determinant of every disease from accelerated aging and heart diseases to cancer (Melnick). Worse it has been known for over a quarter of a century, probably longer than your cardiologist has been practicing. **The good news?** We can get rid of phthalates. We can turn back the hands of time and make our bodies healthier and at the same time get rid of disease. In fact we have to. If we want to reverse diseases and stay healthy, **detoxification is a lifelong pursuit**. Begin with *Detoxify or Die,* and then proceed to the next two books.

Evidence:

- Melnick RL, et al, Mitochondrial toxicity of phthalate esters, *Environ Health Perspect*, 45:51-6, 1982
- Clark K, et al, Observed concentrations in the environment. In: *The Handbook of Environmental Chemistry, Vol 3, Part Q: Phthalate Ester* (Staples CA, ed). New York: Springer, 125-177, 2003
- Vom Saal FS, Welshons WV, Large effects from small exposures. II. The importance of positive controls in low-dose research on bisphenol A, *Environ Res*, 100; 1:50-76, Jan. 2006
- Winberg LD, et al, Mechanism of phthalates-induced inhibition of hepatic mitochondrial B-oxidation, *Toxicology Letters,* 76:63-69, 1995
- Alonso-Magdalena P, et al, The estrogenic effect of bisphenol A disrupts pancreatic B-cell function in vivo and induces insulin resistance, *Environ Health Perspect,* 114:106-12, 2006
- Hurst CH, et al, Environmental phthalates monoesters activate pregnane X receptor-mediated transcription, *Toxicology Applied Pharmacology,* 199:266-74, 2004
- Wolf G, Inhibition of the cellular uptake of folate by blocking synthesis of the membrane and folate receptor, *Nutrition Reviews,* 56; 3 86-87, Mar 1998
- Toda C, et al, Unequivocal estrogen receptor-binding affinity of phthalates esters featured with ring hydroxylation and proper alkyl chain size, *Archives Biochemistry Biophysics,* 431:16-21, 2004
- Takeuchi S, et al, Differential effects of phthalates esters on transcriptional activities via human estrogen receptors A and B, and androgen receptor, *Toxicology,* 210:223-33, 2005
- Lombardo YB, et al, Effects of dietary polyunsaturated n-3 fatty acids on dyslipidemia and insulin resistance in rodents and humans, A review, *J Nutr Biochem,* 17:1-13, 2006

- Alonso-Magdalena P, et al, The estrogenic effect of bisphenol A disrupts pancreatic B-cell function in vivo and induces insulin resistance, *Environ Health Perspect,* 114:106-12, 2006
- Narayanan BA, et al, Docosahexanenoic acid regulated genes and transcription factors inducing apoptosis in human colon cancer cells, *Int J Oncol,* 19:1255-62, 2001
- Jaakkola JJK, et al, The role of exposure to phthalates from polyvinyl chloride products in the development of asthma and allergies: A systematic review and meta-analysis, *Environ Health Perspect,* 116:845-53, 2008
- Turan N, et al, The effect of plasticizers on "sulfate supply" enzymes, *Molecular Cellular Endocrinology,* 244:15-19, 2005
- Seo KW, et al Comparison of oxidative stress and changes of xenobiotic metabolizing enzymes induced by phthalates, *Food Chemical Toxicology,* 42:10 7-114, 2004
- Kim SC, Hong JT, Yun YP, et al, Formation of 8-oxodeoxyguanosine in liver DNA and hepatic injury by peroxisome proliferator clofibrate and perfluorodecanoic acid in rats, *J Toxicol Sci,* 23; 2; 113-119, 1998
- Barr DB, et al, Assessing human exposure to phthalates using monoesters and their oxidized metabolites as biomarkers, *Environmental HealthPerspectives,* 111: 1148-51, 2003
- Campbell SE, et al, Gamma-tocopherol up regulates PPAR gamma expression in SW480 human colon cancer cell lines, *BMC Cancer,* 3; 25:112-25, 2003
- Rogers, SA, Using organic acids to diagnose and manage recalcitrant patients, *Integrative Medicine,* 5; 4:52-61, Aug/Sep 2006
- For hundreds of other references and more details, Rogers, SA, *The Cholesterol Hoax,* prestigepublishing.com

Recognizing the Innocent

Folks continually ask me how they can find a doctor who does this kind of medicine. I am the first to admit it is not easy. This year I'll be asking physician readers of the newsletter to send information if they feel qualified to be in a directory that we would make available. Certainly a doctor who is willing to read something that you ask of him, that pertains to his specialty and your health as his patient, is interested in growing. Many readers are thoroughly disheartened when their physician returns a book unread telling them he doesn't have the time. Would you take your car to a mechanic who "doesn't have time" to read the new manual?? Is you Doctor saying he doesn't have time to grow, to learn? He has no curiosity? He thinks he is so smart that there is nothing else to learn? He is content with the current rate of suffering and death? I have no idea.

On the flip side, at the risk of sounding self-serving, certainly a doctor who encourages you to read something like this book, or displays or sells it in his office shows he is not intimidated by newness and is eager to learn. Furthermore, it indicates he has enough respect for you that he can answer your questions and invite your input. After all, who knows your medical history and the idiosyncrasies of this patient better than you?

We physicians need all the help we can get, for the possibilities of causes are almost endless. One reason I write to educate my patients and readers is so they can become a crucial member of the team. I don't mind at all if they think investigating for a cause in a certain direction seems more indicated, given how they have learned to collate their knowledge of their environmental history, than another route. By understanding the many possibilities of causes, the person involved often has a gut level feeling of which leads we should follow first.

What is the Lame Alibi?

What is the excuse for such flagrant ignorance and neglect of the facts for curing symptoms in medicine? The reality is that the alibi is airtight. **Malpractice is defined not by failing to do what is best, but by not doing what the rest of the herd is doing.** It is as simple as that. And in the books and *TW,* I have given voluminous evidence of how medicine is controlled by the drug industry. Not wanting to bog you down with the politics of medicine here, I have only to remind you of one example from many that tells the story much better. Dr. Marcia Angell, M.D. was the editor of the prestigious *New England Journal of Medicine* for 2 decades. From her front-row seat, she saw first hand how *pharmaceutical marketing* *masquerades as education*, and how *lures, bribes and kickbacks* were so vivid they became the actual titles of chapters in her great book, *The Truth About the Drug Companies* (Random House, New York, 2004).

Clearly only one thing will motivate a physician to learn all this that we were not taught (and still are not) in medical school about how to heal the impossible. He has to have the right ethics. It takes courage to do what is right. Sure it also takes sacrifice, studying, dedication, involves teaching the patient, and bucking the system. But the result is being able to empower folks to heal what now is considered to have no recourse but drugs. As Harry S. Truman said, "The buck stops here." **Pharmacy-focused physicians' slow killing, disguised as modern medical treatment, can only be replaced by the ethical cardiologist who is not afraid to do what is right. God designed the human body to heal, against all odds.**

In this highly sophisticated technological era, we have more than enough tools with which to accomplish right. Instead of $1,500 a year for Lipitor® for cholesterol, a fraction of that buys **Niacin Time** (B3) while the victim finds the underlying cause and finally gets rid of his high cholesterol entirely. Instead of $15,000 a year for Remicade® for rheumatoid arthritis, many have gotten rid of arthritis pain entirely with no drugs by eliminating nightshades (see *Pain Free In 6 Weeks*) and/or doing the macrobiotic diet. Or instead of $150,000 a year for any number of chemotherapy drugs that merely buy a month or so of extended life, the macrobiotic diet has literally cured folks who are alive 10 and 20 years later, drug-free and symptom-free and cancer-free.

Were There Any Accomplices?

You bet there were! Every PFP (pharmacy-focused physician) is guilty of the same crime. Rheumatologists prescribe Remicade® and methyltrexate known to cause cancers, while we and others have published in medical journals (and *Pain Free In 6 Weeks)* how the severest form of arthritis, rheumatoid, can be totally cured in many folks with diets, as one example. Oncologists give drugs they know can kill the heart yet don't give the nutrients that can prevent it (Block), as we've referenced in *TW* for years.

Gastroenterologists major in drugs that turn off gastric secretions that then inhibit nutrient absorption, putting you on a fast track for aging and new diseases, as we showed in *No More Heartburn.* And the psychiatrist drugs everything from depression and OCD to schizophrenia, ADD and even learning disability, and personality disorders. It's almost as though they have forgotten the brain can be a target organ (as we showed in *Depression Cured At Last!),* and instead believe it is merely suffering from a drug deficiency.

The ophthalmologists still tell folks that macular degeneration (that we've literally reversed and cured, and put many of the references in *TW*) is incurable and will lead to blindness. Meanwhile, the diabetologist, pediatrician, allergist, nephrologist and other PFPs are equally guilty of the crime. Sometimes the cure can be as simple as a hidden food or mold allergy (described in *The E.I. Syndrome*).

And I can't imagine being operated on by a surgeon who doesn't want to know my nutrient status first. He has a golden opportunity to find deficiencies that have occurred over a lifetime and correct them. This can markedly improve the chance of surviving the anesthesia without liver and brain damage, not to mention speeding up healing immeasurably (McDaniel). And when physicians from any specialty find folks are multi-drug-resistant, they must get rid of the heavy metals that caused it (Bridges), as described in *The High Blood Pressure Hoax*. They are all accomplices.

Evidence:

- Block KI, et al, Impact of antioxidant supplementation on chemotherapeutic toxicity: a systematic review of the evidence from randomized controlled trials, *International Journal Cancer,* 123:1227-39, 2008
- McDaniel JC, et al, Omega-3 fatty acids effect on wound healing, *Wound Repair Regeneration,* 16:337-45, 2008
- Bridges CC, et al, MRP2 and the DMPS- and DMSA-mediated elimination of mercury and TR- and control rats exposed to thiol s-conjugates of inorganic mercury, *Toxicology Science*, May 28, 2008

How the Cancer Patient is Cheated

I can't leave this book on cardiovascular diseases without again stressing **how often someone with cancer dies not of their cancer, but from a heart killed by chemotherapy.** The tragedy is that many of these same nutrients also protect the heart from chemo death. Why are they not measured or at least used?

The current treatment for cancer lags pathetically behind the science of healing. Let's take a quick look at examples from every aspect. (1) In order to get cancer, you have to have carcinogenic (environmental chemical) damage to genes. But these carcinogens are not sought in conventional medicine, much less gotten rid of.

(2) The same goes for nutrient deficiencies. Many papers over the years, even in high profile journals show that folks, as one mineral example, with higher levels of selenium get fewer cancers. And after they do get them, those with higher levels of selenium have better survival. One of the many mechanisms (because **selenium** is but one mineral in many anti-cancer enzymes) is it **makes cancer cells commit suicide** (called apoptosis) (Hiraoka). If your oncologist doesn't measure your intracellular selenium, how will he know you are not in the top quintile? How will he know to correct this with **SeaSel**?

There are literally hundreds of papers proving the beneficial effects of correcting fatty acids in cancer, yet they are rarely blindly added, but even more rarely measured. As one example, **the right fat-ty acids make cancer cells more vulnerable to chemotherapy** (Pardini). In other words, fatty acid repair makes chemotherapy work better and with fewer side effects. No drug has this advantage.

(3) All chemotherapy induces further nutrient deficiencies, but these are not sought nor corrected. For example, **cisplatin is a frequently used chemotherapy, but causes severe magnesium deficiency** (Hodgkinson). **This in turn leads to cardiomyopathy and death,** or heart attack, or angina, depression, insomnia, exhaustion, migraines, and more. But magnesium is rarely checked and when it is, the wrong inferior serum magnesium is assayed instead of the intracellular erythrocyte or red blood cell magnesium (Whang).

Likewise, **paclitaxel** is one of the most commonly prescribed forms of chemo. It sounds innocent enough, derived from the yew tree bark, but it **causes peripheral neuropathy** in 60% of users. **Vitamin E can inhibit this nasty side effect** (Argyriou), but is rarely prescribed, much less measured. And if it is prescribed, it is not with all 8 forms of vitamin E in a natural supplement, like **E Gems Elite**. For studies (4) show that synthetic nutrients do not work the same as natural ones.

And (5), with vitamin E as an example, when you use only one form of a vitamin like alpha tocopherol or worse, "vitamin E" that is synthetic and lowers the good alpha tocopherol, you suppress the levels of the other 7 parts of real vitamin E, and actually promote cancer. For real vitamin E contains 8 entities, not one. Manufacturers who are proud of their products will give specific details on the package label. This is crucial, for **the wrong supplements can be fertilizer for cancers.**

(6) Glutathione is a major detoxifier the body makes, and is deficient in not only heart patients, but also cancer patients.

That is why it is an integral part of your detox cocktail. To boost **glutathione actually makes chemotherapy work better,** while at the same time it protects the normal cells from the lethal side effect of chemo death (Conklin, Zunino, Smyth). Even though a high percentage of folks die from the side effects of chemotherapy, and glutathione is cheap, available by non-prescription orally, or by prescription if injected, where are the oncologists who measure and correct it? Has it anything to do with the *Wall Street* Journal article that the drugs they routinely prescribe, many of which cost well over $1000 a dose (and that only buy 1-2 months of prolonged life) are sold and administered through their clinics at an obscene 60% mark-up, while glutathione costs less than $2 per injection? (June 2004 *TW*)

(7) Even the **Mayo Clinic showed that cancer patients taking natural supplements live longer than those not taking them** (Jatoi). Not to mention all the references I've given you in previous *TW* proving cancer patients do much better (regardless of whether they choose conventional chemotherapy or not), when their nutritional status is primed with nutrients. **For nutrients had to be low to get the cancer in the first place.** The work of living in this world depletes nutrients daily.

How About Testing Your Oncologist or Other Specialists?

I can't believe some folks put more effort into selecting a new car or stereo/DVD player than the physician who is captain of the ship for their heart or cancer. They would never think of testing him, yet their life depends on it. As one example from our newsletter, *Total Wellness*, nonchalantly ask if he is going to check your HPLA (para-hydroxyl phenyl lactate). If he gives you a blank look or tries to put you down or denigrate the test, you know the answer. It can show cancer, including leukemia is on the move and metastasizing or getting worse long before his conventional tests. It also shows if you need a huge amount of antioxidants, like maybe IV vitamin C, and more. The same can be said for the 8-OHdG

(8-hydroxy-2'-deoxy guanosine) a marker of gene damage also used as a barometer. There are many more tests they probably have never heard of, studied or used, but that are crucial to your survival.

I think a recent article on prostate cancer sums it up beautifully. In "Doctors get more aggressive with prostate cancer" (3D, *The Greenville News*, Oct. 21, 2008) they reported how "watchful waiting" for men with prostate cancer is outdated. It used to be if a guy was 70 they couldn't justify operating because median survival from prostate cancer is 6 years, and average life expectancy was 76. Now that life has been extended to the 80's, they've decided on the new term "active surveillance"! Is that the height of double speak? Sadly urologists still do not measure nutrients proven to stop cancer growth or reprogram the cancer P53 genes back to normal or lower PSA or stop metastases as we've referenced how to in *TW*. It's still the old chemo-hormones-surgery- or -"active surveillance". Such a travesty. What a crime that so many more men will suffer and needlessly die.

Or look at the physicians who prescribe Fosomax® and 1500 mg of calcium a day for osteoporosis. Neither cures it, while that grossly-unbalanced calcium is dumped into arteries to accelerate hardening and aging. Meanwhile they should be tarred and feathered for failing to measure such rudimentary nutrients that are deficient in epidemic proportions, yet crucial for the cure of osteoporosis. I can't believe that there are still physicians who fail to even check vitamins D and K, as well as the minerals and fatty acids needed to make bone! No wonder getting the heavy metals out of bone (that kicked the calcium out in the first place) is beyond their comprehension. And don't even get me started on the biochemical ignorance that is rampant in the pediatric world of autism, learning disability, hyperactivity, bipolar, and ADD!

Bottom line? If I had cancer I would start with the program described in December 2006 *TW,* proven to actually cure cancers when folks who had failed all that medicine has to offer were given as little as 48 hours to live with metastatic cancer, bed-ridden on oxygen. Then get the **Cardio/ION** with an excellent interpretation, as described here.

Clearly it is tremendously logical that **cancer patients should begin with a thorough assessment of their nutrient status**, but it is not standard in medicine. Why? Is it because nutrients do not make nearly the money that drugs do or that it takes biochemical knowledge, or both? If you cannot afford the assay, the nutrients in *The Cholesterol Hoax* cover what vast majorities of folks have been found low in over the last few years. You might want to boost your nutritional levels for a few months with those before considering detoxifying your underlying cancer cause.

Evidence:

- Jatoi A, et al, Is voluntary **vitamin and mineral supplementation associated with better outcome** in non-small cell lung cancer patients? Results from the **Mayo Clinic** cohort, *Lung Cancer,* 49; 1:77-84, Jul 2005
- Hodgkinson E, et al, Magnesium depletion in patients receiving cis-platin-based chemotherapy, *Clin Oncol (R Coll Radiol),* 18; 9:710-8, Nov 2006
- Aggryiou AA, et al, Preventing paclitaxel-induced peripheral neuropathy: a phase II trial of vitamin E supplementation, *J Pain Symptom Manage,* 32; 2:237-44, Sep 2006
- Hiraoka K, et al, Osteosarcoma cell apoptosis induced by selenium, *J Othop Res,* 19; 5:809-14, Sep 2001
- Pardini RS, Nutritional intervention with **omega-3 fatty acids enhances tumor response** to anti-neoplastic agents, *Chem Biol Interact,* 162; 2:89-105, Aug 25, 2006
- Conklin KH, Dietary **antioxidants during cancer chemotherapy**: Impact on chemotherapeutic effectiveness and development of side effects, *Nutr Cancer,* 37; 1:1-18, 2000
- Zunino F, Pratesi G, Sala F, et al, Protective effect of reduced glutathione against cisplatin-induced renal and systemic toxicity and its influence on the therapeutic activity of the antitumor drug, *Chem Biol Interact*, 70: 89-101, 1989
- Smyth JF, Bowman A, Prescott RJ, et al, Glutathione reduces the toxicity and improves quality of life of women diagnosed with ovarian cancer treated with cisplatin: results of the double-blind, randomized trial, *Ann Oncol*, 8:569-73, 1997

Every Age is Affected, Beginning With Neonates

And sadly this information is just as neglected for the newborn and the children who are the future of this planet. As an example, *Environmental Health Perspectives* (Oct 2008), the government's most prestigious journal, shows how fire retardants that were legislated into mattresses damage the brains of newborns. It shows how Teflon, plasticizers, pesticides are just a smattering of the pollutants (all found in the newborn at birth and found in their mattresses) damage not only intellect, but bring on allergies or worse, cancers and other diseases once reserved for the elderly.

Regardless of age, income, intellect, or the number of physician friends you have, you need to get involved for the sake of those you love. *TW* has numerous articles (with references for your physician) that focus on one nutrient at a time, so as to not overwhelm the beginner. As an example, you have learned how **all health hinges on the mitochondria.** In this abbreviated introduction to real medicine, I never even got to tell you that one of the most important minerals in the mitochondria is **Manganese** (not to be confused with magnesium). Nor did I tell you of an organic trace mineral drink so important for boosting scores of crucial trace minerals that you cannot get in isolated form, **IntraMin.** Nor did I tell you about another liquid, **Silicon**, so important for strong cell membranes and for conducting the electricity of life. I fervently recommend a swig of each daily. These are the basic components of youthful cardiac blood vessels, for starters.

But all this and more is in the recommended reading to enable you to take control of your health. To pick and choose, to evaluate what is best for you. Remember, a **disease name or label is nearly inconsequential, meaningless. What matters is what caused it and how you are going to cure it.**

Is There a Cover-Up?

Folks ask me if I feel frustrated by this silent crime in medicine. How can I when others with impeccable credentials have struggled far longer? Harvard's Dr. Kilmer McCully first wrote about homocysteine, *The Homocysteine Revolution*, in 1969, the year I graduated from medical school! He published papers on how homocysteine is such an important risk factor for not only cardiology diseases (four times more prognostic of an early heart attack than high cholesterol), but later on how it can be a harbinger of everything from Alzheimer's, macular degeneration and diabetes to cancer.

Yet to this day in spite of literally hundreds of papers by him and many others on the subject, most cardiologists don't even measure it. Folks continually tell me how when they ask for the test they are told it's not important. If cardiologists do measure it, many only think B12, B6 and folic acid are the remedies. They don't know about NAC, copper, TMG, DHA and many other nutrients that are sometimes the answer to reversing hyperhomocysteinemia (Olszewski). So then Dr. McCully tried a different tack and thought maybe bringing the subject down to a simpler single vitamin like B6 might be easier for physicians (Ellis). No such luck. Forty years later most physicians still don't check for simple homocysteine, much less know all the nutrients that are needed to correct it.

As another very simple example, a few years ago prominent Harvard physicians from the School of Public Health published how the low-fat low cholesterol campaign actually damages health (creating what I call the starving cell membrane). They advised how we should be focusing folks on n-3 fats, the types in **cod liver oil, proven to markedly slash cardiac deaths** (Hu). Yet eight years later how many cardiologists measure and correct omega-3 oils?

Remember decades ago when hotel rooms had no irons, no hair dryers, nor safes, and no Internet connections, now there isn't a hotel room without them. What changed that? The same thing that brought down the Berlin Wall, the thing with the most force: **People Power**. How long will you let this crime go on before you let your doctors and insurance companies know your needs?

So if the folks who are supposed to be leaders in the field of cardiology don't listen to simple advice from medical/research authorities, it will be even longer before physicians realize how important it is to turn off the progression of coronary calcifications diagnosed on ultrafast heartscan with nutrients (Rath, Rogers, Hodis). No, I'm afraid the evidence is clear that the ball is in your court. **Your life depends on you learning** and applying this knowledge while you find a physician who is not blocked, but instead is interested in learning and growing, and helping you (and himself!) live.

Meanwhile, **this is the happiest time of our lives**. Many of us have already cured and witnessed others cure maladies that medicine still insists have "no known cause and no known cure". This is the most optimistic time, for even though we have the greatest challenges, we have more effective tools, backed by decades of selfless research and real-life cures than ever before in the history of man. You control your health.

Evidence:
- Olszewski AJ, McCully KS, **Fish oil decreases serum homocysteine** in hyperglycemic men, *Coronary Artery Disease,* 4:53-60, 1993
- Hu FB, Manson JE, Wilett WC, Types of dietary fat and risk of coronary heart disease: a critical review, *J Am Coll Nutr*, 20; 1:5-19, 2001
- Rath M, et al, **Nutritional supplement program halts progression of early coronary atherosclerosis** documented by ultrafast computed tomography, *J Appl Nutr,* 48:67-78, 1996
- Hodis (cited in previous chapter)
- Ellis JM, McCully KS, **Prevention of myocardial infarction by vitamin B6**, *Res Commun Molec Pathol Pharmacol,* 89; 2:208-220, 1995

Summarizing Your Case

In the next minute while you are reading this, 2 people will die in the U.S. from a heart attack. Is this **epidemic of 2 cardiac deaths every minute** a mere coincidence, or is there an underlying crime? Does being clueless about the evidence constitute being negligent? The universal defense is that a doctor can practice the most inferior medicine and give drugs for every symptom as long as that's what the rest of the pack is doing. Pharmaceutical power and medical politics has herded them away from healing.

Modern medicine fixes every cardiac complaint with drugs (that work by poisoning a biochemical pathway) and surgery (whether stents, bypass or ablation). The result is these don't fix what caused the original malfunction. **In allowing the process to continue to smolder, more damage occurs.** Not to worry, we have another drug. But all the drugs have side effects, top among which are depleting the body of nutrients that it needed to heal. So the victim continues to worsen. But that is chalked up to being expected. After all, he is aging.

The alibi is that this is the way things are done. All the physicians can't be wrong. But who profits from this scheme? The pharmaceutical companies have a shared role in controlling medical education, research, medical boards and societies, insurances, and more. But who is complaining? It is great to have drugs to quickly turn off aggravating symptoms. Who wants to read and have to learn all this difficult stuff!? But shouldn't we reserve drugs for last resort?

Heal? Cure? These are words that you and I have been brainwashed to associate with quackery. They have no place in medicine. Or do they? You have seen a smattering of the decades of research from brilliant folks all over the world who have each dedicated their lives to one particular aspect of the wonderful world within you that is designed to heal. A small army of us has accomplished this curing of "chronic diseases" for decades, but we need more interested physicians to save more folks. The army is too small and getting older.

History shows us that often when ideas such as in this book are presented, the authorities react by first attacking credibility (of physicians, nutrients, etc.), in attempts to destroy or squash the movement. Then after years, they suddenly (re-)discover the very same facts and put them out as though they were new and original. You can't wait that long. We'll all be dead.

The Evidence You Have Before You Demands a Verdict

Now that your life is on the line, it certainly raises a lot of questions:

- Who is guilty of this epidemic of deaths?
- Why has it happened?
- How can we fix it?
- And what is your role in this? For if you don't take charge of your own health now, no one will.

Just remember, you now have your chance to do what is right, just like your cardiologist did... and still does.

Where Does the Evidence Lead You?

By now I know you have figured out "who done it". You know the crime, you know the scene, you know the facts leading up to it, and you know the motive. You know the alibi, and you are armed with overwhelming evidence. You also know the verdict. And more importantly you know you have control over your future so that you are not a victim.

Do you think it's a coincidence that you found this book? For myself, I suffered with over 2 dozen "incurable" illnesses. I had to be brought to my knees before I was blessed with the ability to find the causes and cures. I'm convinced that "All things work together for the good to them that love God, to them who are called **according to his purpose**" (*Romans* 8:28). For it reinforced what I was taught in the *Bible*. When all that high tech medicine has to offer has failed and the patient seemingly has no further options, look at the machinery, the chemistry. For the wonders of the body are analogous to its being like a mini-solar system. The molecular biochemistry continues to prove to us that we were designed to heal, against all odds. As it asks in *I Corinthians*, "Has God not made foolish the wisdom of this world?"

As for you, now that you know medicine's dirty little secret and that you have the power to heal just about anything, what are you going to do with it? For "Everyone to whom much is given, of him will much be required" (*Luke* 12:48). I hope you will go on to save others, beginning with those you love. For if you don't, who will?

Solution Sources

For folks who would like one easy source for all of their nutrients in this book, **NEEDS** carries them (needs.com or 1-800-634-1380).

Item	Web/Company	800#
Daily Detox Drink	happybodies.com	800-HappyBodies
Sencha Premium Organic Green Tea	indigo-tea.com	866-248-3516
Green tea infuser	natural-lifestyle.com	752-2775
Cardio/ION	metametix.com	221-4640
Chelated Manganese, Super DHA	carlsonlabscom	323-4141
SeaSel	intensivenutrition.com	333-7414
IntraMin (71 organic minerals)	druckerlab.com	888-881-2344
Silicon as Ionic Mineral Silica	eidon.com	700-1169

Books and Services
By Sherry A. Rogers, M.D.

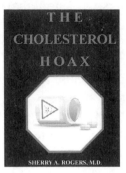

The Cholesterol Hoax

Cholesterol is not the biggest cause of heart disease nor is it predictive of heart disease. In fact, over half the folks who die of a heart attack never had high cholesterol. But they did have other warnings that could have saved their lives, had they been checked. And the cure for these is spelled out here via safe non-prescription nutrients.

Cholesterol is merely the messenger, the smoke detector, alerting you to a curable problem. Why shoot the messenger with a drug when you can find the cause and cure once and for all?

Statin drugs prescribed for high cholesterol poison cholesterol synthesis, which then leads to Alzheimer's, impotence, tooth loss, depression, sudden heart attack, fibromyalgia, chronic fatigue, polyneuropathy, tendon ruptures, insulin resistance, amnesia, suicide, heart failure and cancers, plus statins produce deficiencies of vitamin E, folic acid, and CoQ10, ushering in more diseases and shortening life. Fortunately, there are many non-prescription, cheaper, safer, and more effective agents to control cholesterol damage.

Juicy steaks, cheeses, and wine are not forbidden, but one bite of a more common food ingredient (recommended by dieticians) sends thousands of damaging molecules to every one of your body's trillions of cells and creates high cholesterol. As well, Teflon, plasticizers, PCBs, lead, arsenic, mercury and other unavoidable toxins that we all harbor can trigger coronary artery disease, with or without high cholesterol, as can hidden infections that stem from the teeth, the gut, or former "colds".

Since half the folks who have a heart attack never make it to the hospital in time, you will also learn here how to thwart death with your own home emergency box, plus crucial steps for those who have already survived one. Furthermore, complete with over 700 scientific references for evidence, you will learn more about the prevention and reversal of heart disease than most physicians know, because you need to. For no one can heal you, but you can learn how to heal yourself. Yes, having high cholesterol is one of the luckiest things that ever happened to you, because it led you to this book, which can save your life, regardless of who you are. Clearly, even if you never had high cholesterol you need this book to show you how to thwart the number one cause of death, cardiovascular disease.

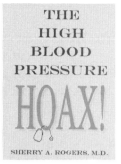

The High Blood Pressure Hoax

Blood pressure drugs guarantee you will get worse, for they actually deplete the nutrients that cause high blood pressure, making sure you will need even more medications as your pressure goes higher and you also develop new symptoms. High blood pressure is not a deficiency of blood pressure-lowering drugs, which also shrink the brain and raise your risk of heart attack, senility, cancer and blindness. But there are dozens of ways you can permanently cure your blood pressure without drugs.

And since healthy blood vessels determine the longevity of every organ in the entire body, **you need this book even if you don't have high blood pressure, for vascular health is key to total body health and longevity.** First of all the health of every single cell of your body depends on the health of your blood vessels that supply them. For example, if you don't want to get Alzheimer's, then you need a healthy brain, but it is only as healthy as its blood supply. Likewise, if you don't want cancer (or you are trying to heal it), it starts (and spreads) in areas of poor circulation. Furthermore, obvious conditions like impotency or erectile dysfunction scream for blood vessel health to be restored.

The High Blood Pressure Hoax will show you that for every ailment, even one as simple as high blood pressure, there are multiple causes and multiple cures. You have a lot to choose from. In fact I would suggest you read the entire book before you chose your program. For by understanding how the various causes work, you (who know your body and medical history better than anyone else) have the optimum opportunity for choosing the best solution for you.

This is the ultimate plan for vascular health, but it doesn't stop there. **This book is also the sequel to the classic, *Detoxify or Die*,** because it takes off from where *DOD* left off, bringing you to even more powerful levels of detoxification. For **it is unprecedented in showing you how to detoxify heavy metals with non-prescription items that are safer, easier, and more efficacious than IV chelation.** Dr. Rogers can't wait to empower you! So let's get started.

161

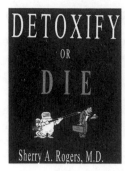

Detoxify or Die

If you don't own this book, you're missing out on the most surefire and thoroughly documented way to heal the impossible and reverse aging, regardless of how "stuck" you might feel. Environmental toxins are ubiquitous, impossible to escape. For example, the phthalates from plastic wrap of foods to Styrofoam trays and cups, plastic bottles for water, soda, juices and infant formula leach into our foods. Once inside our bodies they can create any disease and indefinitely stall the chemistry of healing. EPA studies show this pollutant is in every person and is thousands of times more plentiful than the hundreds of other environmental toxins that insidiously stockpile in the body; taking sometimes decades to produce disease seemingly overnight. Luckily there are a multitude of ways to boost your body's ability to detoxify them, starting with the *Detox Cocktail* that you can make at home every day.

Our lifetime accumulation of pesticides, volatile organic hydrocarbons, heavy metals and more contribute to every disease and symptom. The most exciting part is the proof that **getting rid of environmental toxins reverses diseases for which medicine claims there is no known cause and no known cure!** Contrast this with medicine's solution that consists of a lifetime sentencing to costly medications with a laundry list of side effects. Once you peel away the underlying causes, the body is able to heal itself and disease melts away, as scientific studies in leading medical journals from the Mayo Clinic, for example, clearly prove. **Detoxification is equally crucial for the addicted individual trying to get free from alcohol or addiction to prescription or street drugs.** This is the most thorough program for medical detoxification, including detoxification for folks with infertility and parents-to-be, showing you how to do it safely at home, avoiding the pitfalls. The Resources chapter is complete with where to find everything in this book, 1-800 numbers, addresses, web sites and more, plus over 700 complete scientific references. If you buy only one book this year, make it the classic, *Detoxify or Die.*

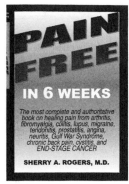

Pain Free in 6 Weeks

All pain has a cause, and once you know the cause, you have the cure. We don't all just look different; we have different chemistries and different underlying causes for our pain.

Old injuries, old age, autoimmune disease, chronic degeneration and even cancer are not the *reasons* for pain. They are mere *labels and excuses* for not finding the true cause and getting rid of it. In fact, the very medications prescribed for pain actually cause deterioration of bone and cartilage, guaranteeing that hip and knee replacement will be needed in the future. And total cure from pain need not be difficult, for the solution may be as simple as eliminating an unidentified food antigen, correcting a nutrient deficiency, healing the gut, or killing an unidentified stealth infection.

For others it has required getting rid of a lifetime's accumulation of everyday toxic chemicals. U.S. EPA studies of chemicals stored in the fat of humans showed that 100% of people harbor environmental chemicals that trigger mysterious back pain, hip pain, arthritis, osteoporosis, painful burning skin, migraines, prostatitis, fibromyalgia, sciatica, degenerating back discs, cystitis, neuropathies, tic doloreau, and even end-stage cancer. When folks get symptoms, they are told that they are a normal consequence of aging, and that there is no known cause or cure. This is totally wrong, as the over 500 scientific references prove. The exciting part is that the majority of folks have total power over their pain. Are you ready to reverse years of pain and become truly **pain free**?

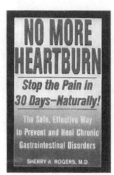

No More Heartburn

The chance of healing any condition in the body is slim to none until the gut is healthy first. Heartburn, indigestion, irritable bowel, spastic colon, colitis, gall bladder disease, gas and bloating are far from benign, for they are all signs of an ailing gastro-intestinal tract. And disease and death began in the gut.

Learn how the many prescription and over-the-counter drugs guarantee that you will not only have worse gut symptoms eventually, but that you can pile on new symptoms, seemingly unrelated to the gut, within the next few years like arthritis, heart problems or cancer.

Come learn how to find the many hidden causes of symptoms like food allergies, Candida overgrowth, Helicobacter, leaky gut, nutrient deficiencies, toxic environment and thoughts, and more. Then learn how to use non-prescription remedies to heal, not merely mask every symptom from mouth to rectum.

Since the gut houses over half the immune system and over half the detoxification system, a silently ailing gut holds back healing any condition indefinitely. This book is also full of new non-prescription Candida and other yeast fighters and protocols, since this is a common unsuspected cause of many diseases.

Learn how **heartburn masked with drugs is a fast road to a heart attack or cancer**, chronic fatigue, chronic pain or fibromyalgia. Explicit clear directions are given for every gut symptom, their causes and cures. For an unhealthy gut is a primary reason for many folks to be stuck at a standstill, unable to heal any further. **If your healing is stalled, chances are you need to start healing the gut first.** You need to heal from the inside out, for **the road to health is paved with good intestines.** (Over 350 references)

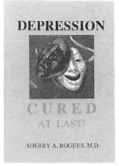

Depression Cured at Last!

Just when you think all has been accomplished, along comes one of the most important books of all. Unique in many ways, (1) it is written for the layperson and the physician, and is appropriate as a medical school textbook. In fact, it should be required reading for all physicians regardless of specialty. (2) It shows that it borders on malpractice to treat depression as a Prozac deficiency, to drug cardiology patients, or any other medical/psychiatric problems without first ruling out proven causes.

With over 700 pages and 1,000 complete references, it covers the **environmental, nutritional** and **metabolic** causes of all disease. It covers leaky gut syndrome, intestinal dysbiosis, hormone deficiencies, hidden sensitivities to foods, molds, and chemicals, dysfunctional detoxification, heavy metal and pesticide poisonings, toxic xenobiotic accumulations, and much, much more.

It is the best blueprint for figuring out what is wrong and how to fix it once and for all. If no one knows what is wrong with you, you need this book. If they know, but say there is no cure, you need this book. If they say you need medications to control your symptoms indefinitely, you need this book. Using depression as an example, it is the protocol for the environmental medicine work-up for all disease: how to systematically find the causes.

It is inconceivable that there is anyone who would not benefit from this book, as it surely leaves drug-oriented medicine in the dust of the 20th century. And it does so by using the only disease that by definition sports a lack of hope. We chose this disease, depression, as a prototype; to be sure to drive home the message that **just when you least expect it, there is always hope. Every symptom has a cause and a cure**. Come learn how to find the causes of yours.

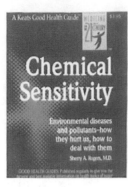

Chemical Sensitivity

This 48-page booklet is the most concise referenced booklet on chemical sensitivity. It is for the person wanting to learn about it, but who is leery of tackling a big book. It is ideal for teaching your physician or convincing your insurance company, as it is fully referenced. And it is a good reference for the veteran who wants a quick concise review.

Most people have difficulty envisioning **chemical sensitivity as a potential cause of everyday maladies.** But the fact is that a lack of knowledge of the mechanisms of chemical sensitivity can be the solo reason that holds many back from ever healing completely. **Some will never get truly well, simply because they do not comprehend the tremendous role chemical sensitivity plays.** For failure to address the role that chemical sensitivity plays in every disease has been pivotal in failure to get well. The principles of environmental controls are of especially vital importance for cancer victims.

If you are not completely well, you need to read this booklet. If you have been sentenced to a lifetime of drugs, whether it is for high blood pressure, high cholesterol, angina, arrhythmia, asthma, eczema, sinusitis, colitis, learning disabilities, chronic pain or cancer, you need this booklet. It matters not what your label is. What matters is whether chemical sensitivity is a factor that no one has explored that is keeping you from getting well. Most probably it is, and this is an inexpensive way to start you on the path toward drug-free wellness. Then give one to your physician and friends who need to learn about pervasive everyday chemicals and their power to cause disease.

The
Scientific Basis
for
Selected
Environmental
Medicine
Techniques

by

Sherry A. Rogers, M.D.

Scientific Basis for Selected Environmental Medicine Techniques contains the scientific evidence and references for the techniques of environmental medicine. It is designed with the patient in mind who is being denied medical payments by insurance companies that refuse to acknowledge environmental medicine.

With this guide a patient may choose to represent himself in small claims court and quote from the book showing, for example, that the *Journal of the American Medical Association* states that "titration provides a useful and effective measure of patient sensitivity". Or he may need to prove to his HMO that a **U.S. Government agency stated, "an exposure history should be taken for every patient"**. Failure to do so can lead to an inappropriate diagnosis and treatment.

It has sections showing medical references of how finding hidden vitamin deficiencies have, for example, enabled people to heal carpal tunnel syndrome without surgery, or heal life threatening steroid-resistant vasculitis, or stop seizures, or migraines, or learning disabilities.

This book is designed for patients who choose to learn how to begin find the causes of their illnesses, rather than merely mask their symptoms with drugs for the rest of their lives. It is also for those who have been unfairly denied insurance coverage, or denied appropriate diagnosis by an HMO that is more concerned about profit than finding the cause of their patients' symptoms. And it is the ideal book with which to educate your PTA, attorney, insurance company, or physicians who still doubt your sanity.

In this era, HMO's tell people what diseases they can have, how long they can have them, and what treatments they can have. And all diseases seem to be deficiencies of drugs, for that is how they are all treated. It is as though arthritis were an Advil deficiency. This book arms you with the ammunition to defend your right to find the causes, get rid of symptoms and drugs, and get reimbursed for it by your insurance company.

167

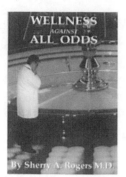

Wellness Against All Odds is the 6th and most revolutionary book by Sherry A. Rogers, M.D. It contains the ultimate healing plan that people have successfully used to beat cancer when they were given 2 weeks, some even 2 days to live by esteemed medical centers. These people had exhausted all that medicine has to offer, including surgery, chemotherapy, radiation and bone marrow transplants. Some had even been macrobiotic failures. And one of the most unbelievable things is that the plan costs practically nothing to implement and most of it can be done at home with non-prescription items.

Of course, in keeping with the other works and going far beyond, this contains the mechanisms of how these principles heal and is complete with the scientific references for physicians. In fact, this program has been proven to more than quadruple cancer survival in the most hopeless forms of cancer (Gonzales, *Nutrition & Cancer*, 33(2): 117-124, 1999).

Did you know, for example, that Harvard physicians have shown how vitamins actually cure some cancers, and over 50 papers in the best medical journals prove it? Likewise, did you know that there are non-prescription enzymes that dissolve cancer, arteriosclerotic plaque, and autoantibodies like lupus and rheumatoid? Did you know that there is a simple inexpensive, but highly effective way to detoxify the body at home to stop the toxic side effects of chemotherapy within minutes? Did you know that this procedure can also reduce chemical sensitivity reactions (from accidental chemical exposures) from 4 days to 20 minutes? Did you know that there are many hidden causes for "undiagnosable" symptoms that are never looked for, because it is easier and quicker to prescribe a pill than find (and fix) the causes?

The fact is that when you get the body healthy enough, it can heal anything. You do not have to die from labelitis. It no longer matters what your label is, from chronic Candida, fatigue, MS, or chronic pain to chemical sensitivity, an undiagnosable condition, or the worst cancer with only days to survive. If you have been told there is nothing more that can be done for you, you have the option of kicking death in the teeth and healing the impossible. Are you game? And **if you can give only one book to a friend with cancer, this is it**.

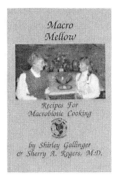

Macro Mellow is a book designed for 4 types of people: (1) For the person who doesn't know a thing about macrobiotics, but just plain wants to cook and eat better to feel better, in spite of the 21st century. (2) It solves the high cholesterol and triglycerides problem without drugs, and is the preferred diet for heart disease patients. In fact, it is the only proven diet to dissolve cholesterol deposits from arterial walls (described in the *Journal of the American Medical Association*, Ornish, 1996). (3) It is the perfect transition diet for those not ready for macro, but needing to get out of the chronic illness rut. (4) It spells out how to feed the rest of the family members who hate macro, while another family member must eat stricter in order to clear "incurable" symptoms.

It shows how to convert the "grains, greens, and beans", strict macro food, into delicious "American-looking" food that the kids will eat. This helps save the cook from making double meals while one person heals. The delicious low-fat whole food meals designed by Shirley Gallinger, a veteran nurse who has worked with Dr. Rogers for over two decades, uses macro ingredients without the rest of the family even knowing. It is the first book to dovetail creative meal planning, menus, recipes and even gardening so the cook isn't driven crazy.

Most likely your kitchen contains a plethora of cookbooks. But you owe it to yourself and your family to learn how to incorporate healing whole foods, low in fat and high in phytonutrients into their diets. **Who you have planning and cooking your meals has been proven to be as important if not more important, than who you have chosen for your doctor.** Medical research has proven time after time the power of whole food diets to heal where high tech medicines and surgery have failed.

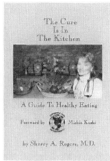

The Cure is in the Kitchen is the next book you should read *after **You Are What You Ate*** to fully understand how to successfully implement the healing macrobiotic diet. It is the first book to ever spell out in detail what all those people ate day to day who cleared their incurable diseases like MS, rheumatoid arthritis, fibromyalgia, lupus, chronic fatigue, colitis, asthma, migraines, depression, hypertension, heart disease, angina, undiagnosable symptoms, and relentless chemical, food, Candida, and electromagnetic sensitivities, as well as terminal cancers.

Dr. Rogers flew to Boston each month to work side by side with Mr. Michio Kushi, as he counseled people at the end of their medical ropes. As their remarkable case histories will show you, nothing is hopeless. Many of these people had failed to improve with surgery, chemotherapy and radiation. Instead their metastases continued to spread. It was only when they were sent home to die within a few weeks that they turned to the diet.

Medical studies confirm that this diet has more than tripled the survival from cancers. And many are documented cures. And the beauty of this diet is that you use God-given whole foods to coax the body into the healing mode. It does not rely on prescription drugs, but allows the individual to heal himself at home.

If you cannot afford a $500 consultation, and you choose not to accept your death sentence or medication sentence, why not learn first hand what these people did and how you, too, may improve your health and heal the impossible.

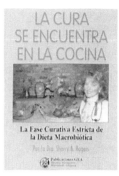

La Fase Curativa Estricta de
la Dieta Macrobiótica

La Cura Se Encuentra En La Cocina

(*The Cure is in the Kitchen* in Spanish)

Este libro explora la relación entre dieta, medio ambiente, salud, y enfermedad y explica como la dieta macrobiótica, basada en cereales integrales, porotos y sus productos y otros alimentos naturales integrales puede prevenir enfermedades y restablecer la salud.

Nos explica cómo una dieta muy artificial contribuye a una variedad de problemas de salud y cómo ciertos aspectos de la vida moderna también nos pueden debilitar.

Un programa macrobiótico consiste de dos fases; pasar gradualmente a una dieta macrobótica o ponerse en una fase curativa estricta de carácter temporario. El objectivo de la fase curativa de esta dieta es aclarar una condición en particular. Es necesariamente, muy estricta e individualizada, y por eso razón, la persona debe consultar un doctor entrenado en la macrobiótica.

Otros libros escritos por Dra. Rogers que tienen que ver con prevenir enfermedades y restablecer la salud son **Cansancio o Intoxicación?, Eres lo que Has Comido,** y **El Síndrome de E.A.**

171

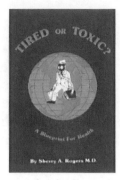

Tired or Toxic? is a 400-page book, and the first book that describes the mechanism, diagnosis and treatment of chemical sensitivity, complete with scientific references. It is written for the layman and physician alike and explains the many vitamin, mineral, essential fatty acid and amino acid analyses that help people detoxify everyday chemicals more efficiently and hence get rid of baffling symptoms, including chronic pain.

It is the first book written for laymen and physicians to describe xenobiotic detoxification, the process that allows all healing to occur. You have heard of the cardiovascular system, you have heard of the respiratory system, the gastrointestinal system, and the immune system. But **most have never heard of the chemical detoxification system, which is the main determinant of whether we have chemical sensitivity, cancer, and in fact, every disease.**

This program shows you how to diagnose and treat many resistant everyday symptoms and use molecular medicine techniques. It also gives the biochemical mechanisms in easily understood form, of how Candida creates such a diversity of symptoms and how the macrobiotic diet heals "incurable" end stage metastatic cancers. It is a great book for the physician you are trying to win over, and shows you how chemical sensitivity masquerades as common symptoms. It then explores the many causes and cures of chemical sensitivity, chronic Candidiasis, brain fog or toxic encephalopathy, and other "impossible to heal" medical labels.

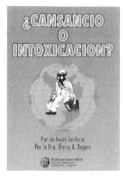

Cansancio o Intoxicacion?
(*Tired or Toxic?* in Spanish)

El lego informado reconoce que a medida que el mundo se vuelve más tecnológico, el hombre pierde proporcionalmente más control sobre su vida. Este libro le permitirá recuperar el control de su salud, ofreciéndole mayor capacidad para formar equipo con su medico para diagnosticar y tratar su condición.

Esta información es vitalmente importante ahora ya que a todos toca con cualquier síntoma tal como la sensibilidad química, alto colesterol, fatiga crónica, complejo relacionado a Cándida, depresion, Alzheimer, hipertensión, diabetes, enfermedad cardíaca, osteoporosis y más.

Dra. Rogers se encuentra en la avanazada de la educación pública sobre los efectos del medio ambiente en el individuo.

Otros libros escritos por Dra. Rogers que tienen que ver con prevenir enfermedades y restablecer la salud son **Eres lo que Has Comido, El Síndrome de E.A.,** y **La Cura Se Encuentra En La Cocina:** La Fase Curativa Estricta de la Dieta Macrobiotica.

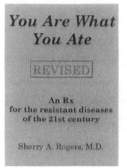

You Are What You Ate

This book is indispensable as the primer and introduction to the macrobiotic diet. The macrobiotic diet is the specialized diet with which many have healed the impossible, including end-stage metastatic cancers. This is after medicine had given up on them and they had been given only months or weeks to live. Yes, they have rallied after surgery, chemotherapy and radiation had failed. Life was seemingly, hopelessly over, yet they kicked death in the teeth.

Understandably, this diet has also enabled many chemically sensitive universal reactors, and highly allergic and even "undiagnosable people" to heal. It has also enabled those to heal who had "wastebasket" diagnostic labels such as chronic fatigue, fibromyalgia, MS (multiple sclerosis), rheumatoid arthritis, depression, chronic infections, colitis, asthma, migraines, lupus, chronic Candidiasis, sarcoidosis, neuropathies, and much more.

Although there are many books on macrobiotics, this is one that takes the special needs of the allergic person and those with multiple food and chemical sensitivities as well as chronic Candidiasis into account. It provides details and case histories that the person new to macrobiotics needs before he embarks on the strict healing phase, as meticulously described in the sequel, *The Cure is in the Kitchen*.

Even people who have done the macrobiotic diet for a while will find reasons why they have failed and tips to improve their success. When a diet such as this has allowed many to heal their cancers, any other condition "should be a piece of cake".

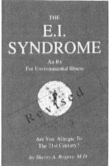

The E.I. Syndrome, Revised is a 635-page book that is necessary for people with **environmental illness.** It explains chemical, food, mold allergies, and Candida sensitivities, nutritional deficiencies, testing methods and how to do the various environmental controls and diets in order to get well.

Many docs buy this by the hundreds and make them mandatory reading for patients, as it contains many pearls about getting well that are not found anywhere else. In this way it increases the fun of practicing medicine, because patients are on a higher educational level and office time is more productive for more sophisticated levels of wellness. It covers hundreds of facts that make the difference between E.I. victims versus E.I. conquerors. It helps patients become active partners in their care and thereby get better results, while avoiding doctor burnout. It covers the gamut of the diagnosis and treatment of environmentally induced symptoms.

Because the physician author was a severe universal reactor who has recovered, this book contains mountains of clues to wellness. As a result, many have written that they healed themselves of resistant illnesses of all types by reading this book. This is in spite of the fact that no consulted physicians were able to diagnose or effectively treat them. If you are not sure what causes your symptoms, this, Dr. Rogers' very first book, is a great start.

Many veteran sufferers have written that they had read many books on aspects of allergy, chronic Candidiasis and chemical sensitivity and thought that they knew it all. Yet (they wrote that) what they learned *in **The E.I. Syndrome, Revised*** enabled them to reach that first pinnacle of wellness.

Total Wellness Newsletter

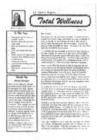 For over a decade and a half, this referenced monthly newsletter has kept folks and physicians up to date on new findings. Since Dr. Rogers is constantly researching, lecturing around the globe, maintaining a private practice of 38 years, doing television and radio shows, writing for health magazines and physicians, and has published over 20 scientific papers and over 15 books in 20 years, she is pedaling as fast as she can.

There is literally an avalanche of new information, but we don't want you to have to wait for a new book on the subject to learn about it or worse, wait decades for it to reach the media or your doctor. We want that practical and useful instruction in your hands this month. For example, TW 2005-9 tells of a device that is three times less expensive, easier and more effective than the one in "Pain Free In 6 Weeks",

Furthermore, the field of environmental medicine, because it is so all encompassing, can be overwhelming at times. So in addition to bringing you the new, we also focus on the overall perspective and the practical solutions you can do today.

In this era, because we cannot get the information out to you fast enough, we use the newsletter as our communication link. **By sending you to the medical school of the future each month,** *Total Wellness* **will teach you useful facts years before they will be presented elsewhere, and it is practical and action-oriented, giving you explicit directions and sources.** For pennies a day you really cannot afford to be without this life-altering unique information.

We continually receive kind letters that read, "I had to laugh last week when all the newspapers and television shows were abuzz with that hot new medical discovery. If they had been readers of your newsletter, they could have learned about it 10 years ago, as I did!"

Non-Patient Phone Consultations
With Dr. Sherry A. Rogers

Many people are stuck. They have an undiagnosable condition, or they have a label but have been unable to get well. Or they have a "dead-end" label that means nothing more can be done. These people could benefit from a non-patient consultation with Dr. Rogers to explore what diagnostic and treatment options may exist that they or their health care providers are not aware of. For this reason we offer prepaid, scheduled phone consultations with the doctor. Call her office, 315-488-2856 for more information. It is a good idea to read at least two of her latest books and a couple of years of the TW newsletter in order to help you ask more informed questions that will save you money and time.

Many schedule for interpretation by Dr. Rogers of their Cardio/Ion and other laboratory data. The molecular biochemistry of healing plus reversal of environmental pollutants have evolved into a new medical specialty. Healing hinges on the knowledge which goes far beyond mere checking of what lies outside the "normal range" or using computer generated suggestions.

Make sure to include your recent medical reports from the last few years, as this promotes more precise tailoring of biochemical parameters to your individual case.

PRESTIGE PUBLISHING
1-800-846-6687
www.prestigepublishing.com

Price List

Books
Is Your Cardiologist Killing You?	$19.95
The Cholesterol Hoax	$23.95
The High Blood Pressure Hoax	$19.95
Detoxify or Die	$22.95
Pain-Free In 6 Weeks	$19.95
No More Heartburn	$15.00
Depression Cured At Last!	$24.95
Chemical Sensitivity (booklet)	$ 3.95
The Scientific Basis for Environmental Medicine Techniques	$17.95
Wellness Against All Odds	$17.95
Macro Mellow	$12.95
The Cure Is In The Kitchen	$14.95
Tired or Toxic?	$18.95
You Are What You Ate	$12.95
The E.I. Syndrome Revised	$17.95

Spanish Translations
Cansancio o Intoxicacion?	$30.00
La Cura Se Encuentra En La Cocina	$30.00

Total Wellness Newsletter
Monthly referenced newsletter on current wellness and
healing information
Current 1 year subscription (12 issues, 8 pages, referenced)	$54.00
Back issues/1 year (12 issues)	$36.00
Individual back issues	$ 8.00

Non-Patient Phone Consultations
Telephone consultations are available with Dr. Rogers.
For scheduling information, contact Dr. Rogers' office at (315) 488-2856.

Radio Shows

Here are a few examples of where you can often hear Dr. Rogers live and call in with questions, also these shows often are available on tape, CD, or archived on the net for weeks after the show. And you can contact them to ask for future shows with Dr. Rogers

www.kbjs.org
www.hwwshow.com
www.radiomartie.com
www.tantalk1340.com
www.frankieboyer.com
www.thepowerhour.com
www.ksevradio.com or .hotzehwc.com

To have Dr. Rogers speak at your local hospital, church, or organization, contact: orders@prestigepublishing.com

Scientific papers published by Sherry A. Rogers, M.D., in medical journals and medical newspapers:

Rogers, SA, Using organic acids to diagnose and manage recalcitrant patients, *Integrative Medicine*, 5; 4:52-61, Aug/Sep 2006 (physician readers receive 1.5 CME credits for completing quiz)

Rogers, SA, Using organic acids to diagnose and manage recalcitrant patients, *Alternative Therapies*, 12; 4:44-53, July/August 2006 (physician readers receive 1.5 CME credits for completing quiz)

Rogers, SA, Lipoic acid as a potential first agent for protecting from and treatment of mycotoxicosis, *Arch Environ Health*, 58; 8:528-32, Aug. 2004

Rogers SA, Solonaceae (Nightshade) sensitivity as a reversible cause of juvenile and adult rheumatoid arthritis, chronic degenerative disc pain, and osteoarthritis, *Journal of Applied Nutrition* 52; 1:2-11, 2002

Rogers SA, Childhood asthma: Causes and cures, *Journal Southeastern Society Pediatric Dentistry*, 8; 4:16-18, 2002

Rogers SA, Understanding the causes and cures of childhood diseases-Part I, *Journal Southeastern Society Pediatric Dentistry*, 8;4: 26-28, 2002

Rogers SA, Diagnosing the tight building syndrome, *Environmental Health Perspectives*, 1987; 76:195-98 (This is the main scientific publication of the U.S. government's National Institutes of Health.)

Rogers SA, Indoor fungi as part of the cause of recalcitrant symptoms of the tight building syndrome, *Environment International,* 17; 4:271-2765, 1991 (journal goes to 152 countries)

Rogers SA, Unrecognized magnesium deficiency masquerades as diverse symptoms, evaluation of an oral magnesium challenge test, *International Clinical Nutrition Reviews*, 11; 3:126-130, July 1991

Rogers SA, A case of atopy with inability to form IgG, *Annals of Allergy,* 43; 3:165-166, Sept 1979

Rogers SA, A thirteen month work, leisure, and sleep environmental fungal survey, *Annals of Allergy*, 50:37-40, Jan 1983

Rogers SA, A comparison of commercially available mold survey services, *Annals of Allergy*, 50; 37-40, Jan 1983

Rogers SA, In-home fungal studies, methods to increase the yield, *Annals of Allergy*, 49; 35-37, July 1982

Rogers SA, Zinc deficiency as a model for developing chemical sensitivity, *International Clinical Nutrition Reviews,* 10; 1:253-259, Jan 1990

Rogers, SA, Diagnosing the tight building syndrome or diagnosing chemical hypersensitivity, *Environment International,* 15; 75-79, 1989

Rogers SA, Resistant cases, Response to mold immunotherapy and environmental and dietary controls, *Clinical Ecology, Archives for Human Ecology in Health and Disease*, 5; 3:115-120, 1987/88

Rogers SA, Diagnosing chemical hypersensitivity: Case examples, *Clinical Ecology* 6; 4:129-134, 1989

Rogers SA, Provocation-Neutralization of cough and wheezing in a horse, *Clinical Ecology*, 5; 5:185-187, 1987/88

Rogers SA, Is it chronic low back pain or environmental illness?, *Journal of Applied Nutrition*, 46:106-109, Nov. 4, 1994

Rogers SA, Improvement in chemical sensitivity with the macrobiotic diet, *Journal of Applied Nutrition*, 48; 3:85-93, 1997

Rogers SA, Is your cardiologist killing you?, *Journal of Orthomolecular Medicine*, 8;2:89-97, 1993

Rogers SA, How the sick get sicker by following current medical protocol: The example of undiagnosed magnesium deficiency, *J Orthomolecular Medicine*, 11; 2:63-68, 1996

Rogers SA, A practical approach to the person with suspected indoor air quality problems, *Internat Clin Nutr Rev*, 10; 1:253-9, Jan 1990

Rogers SA, Chemical sensitivity; Breaking the paralyzing paradigm, Part I, *Internal Medicine World Report*, 7; 4:1, 15-17, Feb 1-15, 1992

Rogers SA, Chemical sensitivity: Breaking the paralyzing paradigm, Diagnosis and treatment, Part II, *Intern Med World Rep*, 7; 6:2, 21-31. Mar 1-15, 1992

Rogers SA, Chemical sensitivity: Breaking the paralyzing paradigm. How knowledge of chemical sensitivity enhances the treatment of chronic diseases, Part III, *Intern Med World Rep*, 7; 8:13-16, 32-33, 40-41, Apr 15-30, 1992

Rogers SA, Letters to the editor, *Intern Med World Rep*, May 1-15, 1992

Rogers SA, When stumped, think environmental medicine, *Intern Med World Rep* 7; 13:3, July 1992

Rogers SA, Is it senility or chemical sensitivity?, *Intern Med World Rep*, 7;13:3, July 1992

Rogers SA, How cost effective is improving the work environments?, *Intern Med World Rep*, 7;14:48, Aug 1992

Rogers SA, Is it recalcitrant arrhythmia or environmental illness?, *Intern Med World Rep*, 7;19:28, Nov 1-14, 1992

(Rogers SA (ed.), Chester AC, Sick building syndrome and the nose, *Intern Med World Rep*, 8:4:25-27, Feb 1993)

Scientific presentations in major international indoor air symposia, also published in their respective proceedings:

1. Rogers SA, A practical approach to the person with suspected Indoor air quality problems, *The 5th International Conference on Indoor Air Quality and Climate*, Toronto, **Canada**, Canada Mortgage and Housing Corporation, Ottawa, Ontario, vol. 5:345-349, 1990

2. Rogers SA, Diagnosing the tight building syndrome, in intradermal method to provoke chemically induced symptoms, *Man and His Ecosystem, Proceedings of the 8th World Clean Air Congress 1989,* Brasser LJ, Mulder WC, eds, The Hague, Netherlands, Society for Clean Air in The Netherlands, P.O. Box 186, 2600 AD Delft, **The Netherlands,** vol 1:199-204, 1989

3. Rogers SA, Case studies of indoor air fungi used to clear recalcitrant conditions, *Healthy Buildings '88*, CIB Conference in Stockholm, Sweden, Sept 1988, Swedish Council for Building Research, **Stockholm,** Eds: Berglund S, Lindvall T, Mansson LG, p 127, 1988

5. Rogers SA, Diagnosing the tight building syndrome, Indoor Air '87, *Proceedings of the 4th International Conference on Indoor Air Quality and Climate,* West Berlin, Seifert B, Esdorn H, Fischer M, Ruden H, Wegner J, eds., Institute for Water, Soil and Air Hygiene, D 1000, **Berlin,** 33, vol 2:772-776, Aug 1987

6. Rogers SA, Indoor air quality and environmentally-induced illness, A technique to reverse chemically-induced symptoms, in patients, *Proceedings of the ASHRAE Conference, Indoor Air Quality '86, Managing Indoor Air for Health and Energy Conservation*, p 71-77, 1986, ASHRAE American Society for Heating, Refrigeration and Air Conditioning Engineers), 1791 Tullie Circle, NE, **Atlanta** GA, 30329

7. Also listed in the **EPA's** *Indoor Air Reference Bibliography*,
United States Environmental Protection Agency, *Indoor Air, Reference Bibliography*, EPA/600/8-89/067F, July 1989; IND-1501 and IND-2701 (pg c81 and c162), Office of Health and Environmental Assessment, **Washington**, DC 20460

Summary of Product Sources

Chapter 1
- Cardio/ION, ADMA, metametrix.com, 1-800-221-4640
- Natural Lifestyle, natural-lifestyle.com, 1-800-752-2775
- Cod Liver Oil, E Gems Elite, Chelated Magnesium, Arginine Powder, Solar D Gems 2000, carlsonlabs.com, 1-800-323-4141
- PhosChol, nutrasal.com, 1-800-777-1886
- Natural Calm, supervites.net, 1-888-800-1180
- Magnesium Chloride Solution, windhampharmacy.com, 518-734-3033
- DMSA, vrp.com, 1-800-877-2447
- Captomer, Perfusia, needs.com, 1-800-634-1380
- The High Blood Pressure Hoax, prestigepublishing.com, 1-800-846-6687

Chapter 2
- Niacin-Time, Super DHA, Cod Liver Oil, carlsonlabs.com, 1-800-323-4141
- Policosanol, protherainc.com, 1-888-488-2488
- E Gems Elite, Tocotrienols, Gamma Tocopherol, carlsonlabs.com, 1-800-323-4141
- HDL Rx, integrativeinc.com, 1-800-931-1709
- Q-ODT, intensivenutrition.com, 1-800-333-7414
- PhosChol, nutrasal.com, 1-800-777-1886

Chapter 3
- Cod Liver Oil, E Gems Elite, carlsonlabs.com, 1-800-323-4141
- Gamma E Gems, ACES w/ Zinc, carlsonlabs.com, 1-800-323-4141
- R-Lipoic Acid, SeaSel, Q-ODT, intensivenutrition.com, 1-800-333-7414
- PhosChol, nutrasal.com, 1-800-777-1886
- Magnesium Chloride Solution (Rx), windhampharmacy.com, 518-734-3033
- Natural Calm, supervites.com, 1-888-800-1180
- Super Milk Thistle, integrativeinc.com, 1-800-931-1709
- Mag Chlor 85, painstresscenter.com, 1-800-669-CALM
- Cardio/ION, metametrix.com, 1-800-221-4640
- Comprehensive Stool Test, Doctor's Data, 1-800-323-2784
- Kyolic Liquid, Kyo-Chrome, kyolic.com, 1-800-421-2998
- Abx Support, protherainc.com, 1-888-488-2488
- Nattokinase, allergyresearchgroup.com, 1-800-545-9960

Chapter 4
- Vitamin B1 (100 mg), E Gems Elite, carlsonlabs.com, 1-800-323-4141

- Gamma E Gems, Solar D Gems, carlsonlabs.com, 1-800-323-4141
- Acetyl L-Carnitine Powder, carlsonlabs.com, 1-800-323-4141
- Cardio/ION, Porphyrin, Heavy-Metal Provocation, metametrix.com, 1-800-221-4640
- Corvalen (D-Ribose), integrativeinc.com, 1-800-931-1709
- Q-ODT (sublingual Coenzyme Q10), Ananase, intensivenutrition.com, 1-800-333-7414
- Far infrared sauna, hightechhealth.com, 1-800-794-5355
- Far infrared sauna, saunaray.com, 1-877-992-1100
- Zinc Balance, jarrow.com, 1-800-634-1380
- Lumen, lumenphoton.com, 1-828-863-4834

Chapter 5
- Solar D Gems, Vitamin K2, Super DHA, Arginine Powder, E-Gem Elite, Gamma E Gems, Tocotrienols, Cod Liver Oil, Fish Oil, carlsonlabs.com, 1-800-323-4141
- Cardio/ION, metametrix.com, 1-800-221-4640
- Kyolic Liquid, kyolic.com, 1-800-421-2998
- NSC-24 Beta Glucan Circulatory Formula, nsc24.com, 1-888-541-3997
- SeaSel, intensivenutrition.com, 1-800-333-4141
- PhosChol, nutrasal.com, 1-800-777-1886
- Super Milk Thistle X, integrativeinc.com, 1-800-931-1709

Chapter 6
- Daily Detox Drink, happybodies.com, 1-800-HAPPYBODIES
- Sencha Premium Organic Green Tea, indigo-tea.com, 1-866-248-3516
- Green tea infuser, natural-lifestyle.com, 1-800-752-2775
- Cardio/ION, metametix.com, 1-800-221-4640
- Chelated Manganese, Super DHA, carlsonlabs.com, 1-800-323-4141
- SeaSel, intensivenutrition.com, 1-800-333-7414
- IntraMin, druckerlabs.com, 1-888-881-2344
- Silicon, eidon.com, 1-800-700-1169